UNIVERSITY OF
Cincinnati
COLLEGE OF
Nursing

UNIVERSITY OF
Cincinnati
COLLEGE OF
Nursing

125 YEARS OF TRANSFORMING HEALTH CARE

WENDY HART BECKMAN, M.A.

ORANGE *frazer* PRESS
Wilmington, Ohio

ISBN 9781939710208

Published for the University of Cincinnati by:
Orange Frazer Press
P.O. Box 214
Wilmington, OH 45177
Telephone: 800.852.9332 for price and shipping information.
Website: *www.orangefrazer.com*
www.orangefrazercustombooks.com

Book and cover design: Brittany Lament and Orange Frazer Press
All photos courtesy of the University of Cincinnati unless otherwise noted.

Library of Congress Control Number 2014951257

Printed in the United States of America
First edition, first printing

http://nursing.uc.edu/events/125th-anniversary.html
Visit the 125th Anniversary website to view a complete archive of class photos, videos and the Legacy Award recipients.

To all past, present and future University of Cincinnati College of Nursing
faculty, staff, students and alumni who ensure that our patients receive exquisite,
patient-centered, holistic, culturally competent care.

Be it Proclaimed:

Whereas, The University of Cincinnati College of Nursing has been a leader in nursing education and the transformation of health care since its founding 125 years ago; and

Whereas, The UC College of Nursing has made history by offering the nation's first baccalaureate program in nursing in 1916 and in 1956 became one of the first colleges to offer a master's of science in nursing (MSN) degree; and

Whereas, The UC College of Nursing has built a reputation of quality education since 1942, when they became a charter member of the National League for Nursing, the national accrediting agency, and has maintained accreditation without interruption; and

Whereas, The UC College of Nursing has grown to offer a wide range of educational pathways and outstanding research, in order to meet the needs of the community. These include online, onsite, and hybrid offerings including the Bachelor of Science in Nursing program, RN to BSN completion program, Accelerated graduate program, Nurse Educator certificate program, Master of Science in Nursing program with multiple specialties, Post-Master's certificate programs and doctoral programs in nursing practice and nursing science; and

Whereas, The UC College of Nursing, with nearly 3,000 current students, has been a collaborative educator of nursing leaders who serve the local Cincinnati community, the State of Ohio, as well as, national and international populations; and

Whereas, The UC College of Nursing has been an early adopter of technology in order to expand reach and access to nursing education and health care provision through the creative leveraging of technology, in partnership informed by the community they serve.

Now, Therefore, I, John Cranley, Mayor of the City of Cincinnati do hereby proclaim November 8, 2014, as "University of Cincinnati College of Nursing Day" in Cincinnati.

WHAT WE STAND FOR

Vision

Through creative leveraging of technology, the UC College of Nursing will
lead the transformation of health care in partnership informed by the people we serve.

Mission

Develop nurse leaders who are empowered to generate, explore and
apply nursing knowledge for evolving health care environments.

Core Values

Collaboration

Accountability

Integrity

Respect

Excellence

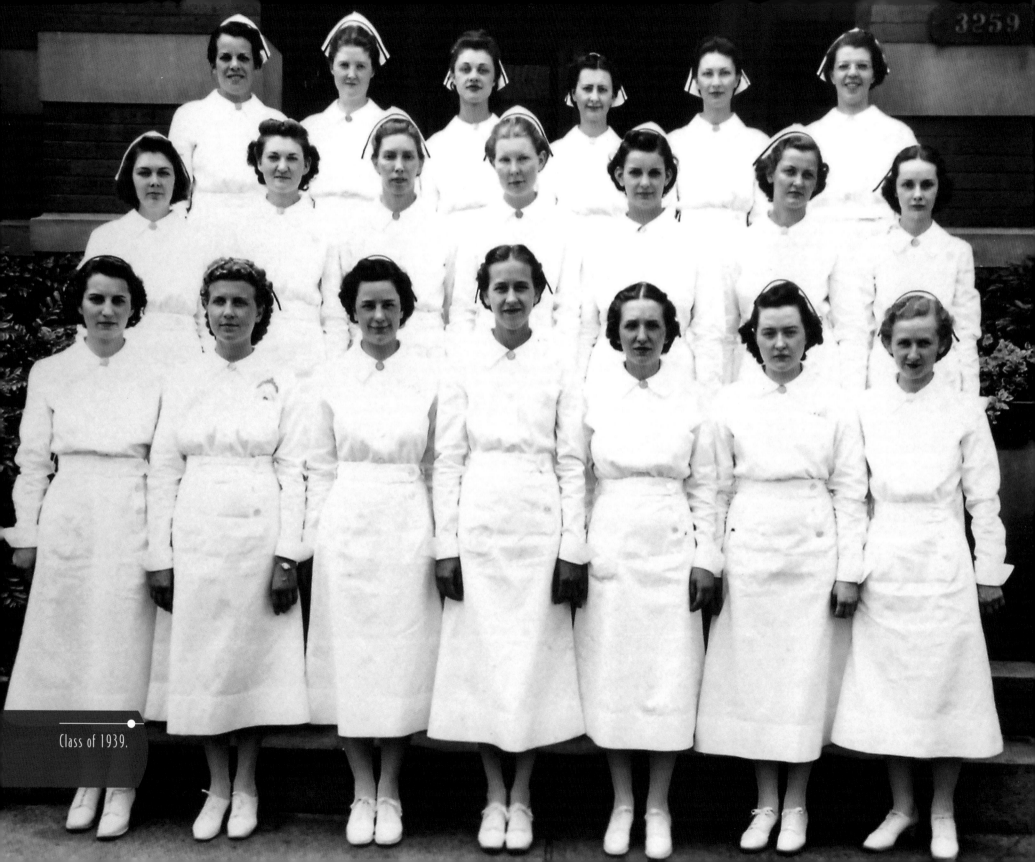

Class of 1939.

ACKNOWLEDGMENTS

August 2014

First and foremost, Jean Brim Cahall, RN, BSN, MSN, EdD, must be acknowledged for her exhaustive efforts in creating the *Pictorial History of the College of Nursing & Health, University of Cincinnati, 1889–1989*. Published for the college's centennial, the volume provided detailed documentation of the life of the college through its students, faculty and administration, as well as the setting in which they operated. It proved to be a valuable resource for this current volume. While Dr. Cahall described the foundations of the past of the University of Cincinnati (UC) College of Nursing, this volume will bring the readers up to date regarding the many changes of the last 25 years and give them a glimpse into where the UC College of Nursing (CON) is going in the future.

I thank the people who gave me their time for interviews. One of those was Jean Wedbush who with her husband, Ed, generously support the college. I asked her if there was one most poignant memory from her days as a registered nurse. At first she said, "not really" because there were so many, but then she quickly corrected herself and said, "Working on pediatrics at night. I had a lot of opportunity to be comforting." Dean Glazer then immediately shared that she had been hospitalized as a child, how frightening it had been, and how much comfort the nurses had provided her in the night.

What I then saw, as I looked at these two strong women, sitting across the table from one another, was—yes, a generous donor and the dean of the recipient college—but even more than that, I saw a registered nurse whose most meaningful memory was comforting scared children, and a woman who was at one time a scared child who was comforted by the nurses. A girl who then went on to pave the way for other children to become nurses who could comfort children in the night. And then do so much more.

I also thank Melanie Cannon in the CON Department of Marketing and Shelley Johnson in the CON Office of Development for their great assistance. Without them, this project could not have succeeded.

Finally, the publication of this book was sponsored in part through the generous support of the Betty J. Michael Historical Preservation Fund (Betty Shewalter, BSN '46) and numerous other alumni and friends of the UC College of Nursing. Without their dedicated commitment, this book would not exist.

—*Wendy Hart Beckman, MA*

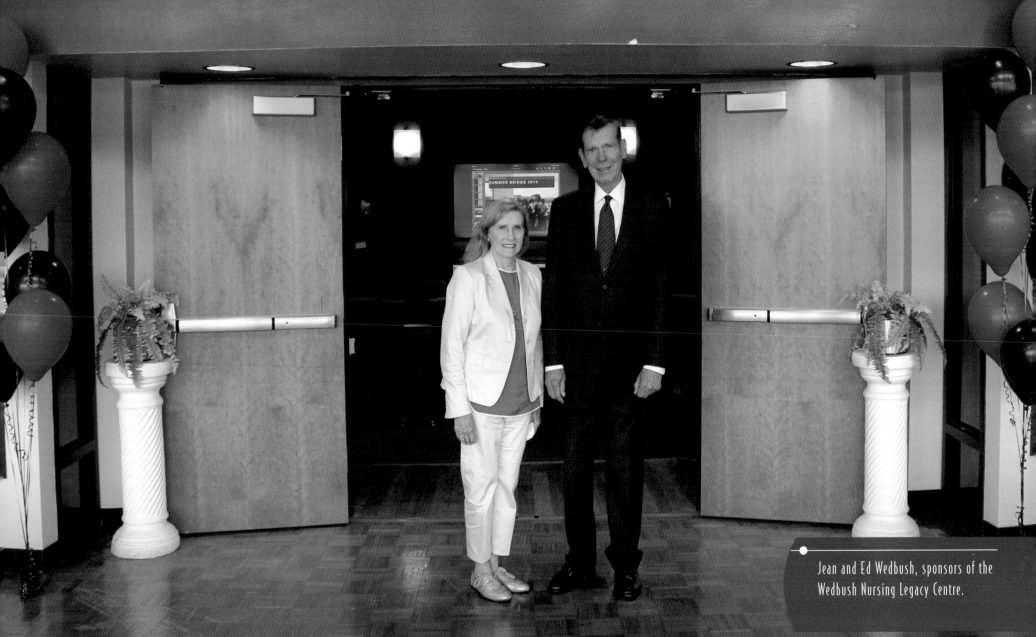

Jean and Ed Wedbush, sponsors of the Wedbush Nursing Legacy Centre.

FOREWORD

"UC Nurses. We See Leaders." That's the concept that inspires our University of Cincinnati College of Nursing today. One hundred and twenty-five years ago, that same kind of leadership existed among the founders who first formed the college as a training school for nurses.

At that time, the first nursing schools were taking shape as our society began to understand the role of germs in disease and to embrace the need for cleanliness. Today we have almost come to take nursing for granted because they are indispensable to the health care system. Their role has dramatically changed and grown. But anyone who has been hospitalized or experienced health issues recognizes the profoundly important role that the nurse plays in our health and well-being.

We are grateful to our predecessors who had the vision to create a formal nursing education program, and at the University of Cincinnati we take great pride in what their vision has become today. In its earliest days, the founders understood the need for nursing students and educators to work closely with a hospital, and that relationship between pedagogy and real-life health care continues stronger than ever.

Our College of Nursing develops new nurses, health care practitioners, nursing educators, nurse administrators and researchers not only for our region and state, but for an impact across the country and around the world. As a full partner in the range of disciplines available at our Academic Health Center, the College of Nursing remains a true leader. And for the many future generations who will follow us, we will work tirelessly to make sure it continues to do so.

Santa J. Ono, PhD
President, University of Cincinnati

Beverly Davenport, PhD
Senior Vice President for Academic Affairs and Provost

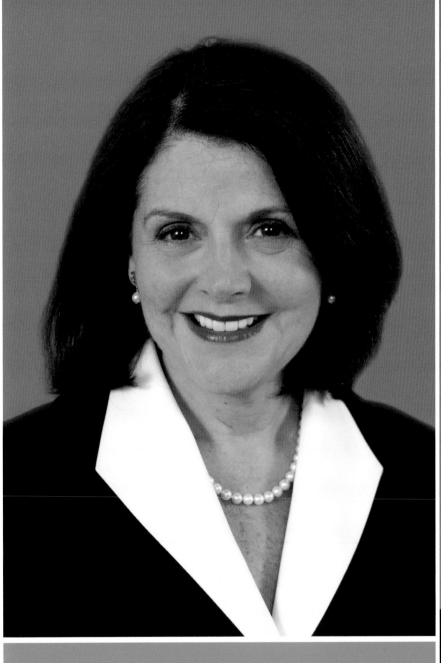

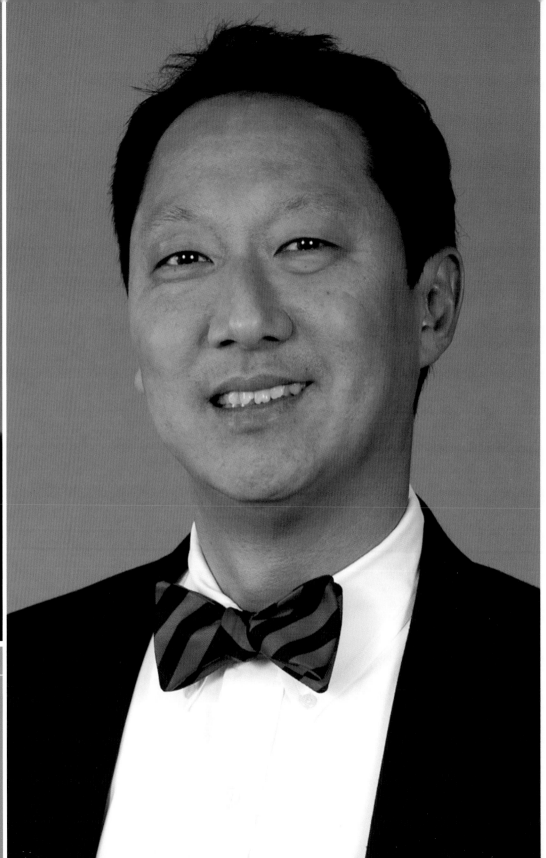

Top: Senior Vice President for Academic Affairs and Provost
Beverly Davenport, PhD
Right: University of Cincinnati President, Santa J. Ono, PhD

INTRODUCTION

Growing up as a child of a physician and a nurse, I was acutely aware of these health care professions and their impact and rewards. As I became destined to be part of the field myself, I experienced the demands, the challenges and the changes that were occurring in the way care was provided, managed and led. Even with that awareness, it was hard to imagine the drastic transformation that health care, and more specifically, nursing would undergo over the years to come.

As I reflect on the history of the University of Cincinnati College of Nursing and the nursing profession, the significant progress that we have undergone amazes me. In 1889, a powerful decision was made in Cincinnati—to open the doors of the Cincinnati Training School for Nurses. This decision, which positively changed health care in the city, led to an institution that has become a leader in nursing education, not just in Cincinnati, but also nationally and globally. Now, 125 years later, nursing itself has become the backbone of health care across the nation. Our college continues to grow and evolve daily.

When I read through the list of the esteemed men and women who worked to open our doors, I can't help but wonder if they had any idea of the impact they were making on the future of health care. I applaud them and thank them for believing in the promise of nursing education. I hope that they continue to serve as an example for nurses and non-nurses alike of the difference our financial and personal support and efforts can have on the future.

As our program grew into existence, hospitals in the city relied upon our first graduates to not only nurse the sick, but to cook and clean—tasks that at the time were instrumental in improving nutrition and cleanliness. In time, the nursing profession expanded to embrace three main tenets—education, research and practice. It transformed from processes and tasks to a science built upon critical thinking and discovery. Just as Florence Nightingale had done before us, nurses took on a crucial role in the improvement of processes, the implementation of technology and the discovery of knowledge.

Today, we continue to innovate in the areas of education, research and practice.

However, this change in the profession was not a series of coincidences. To get at the heart of our transformation, one must look at the heart of our college—our alumni. As the current dean, I have had the pleasure to meet with alumni across the country. Each visit reinforces my commitment and pride in our college, as I get to know the strong women and

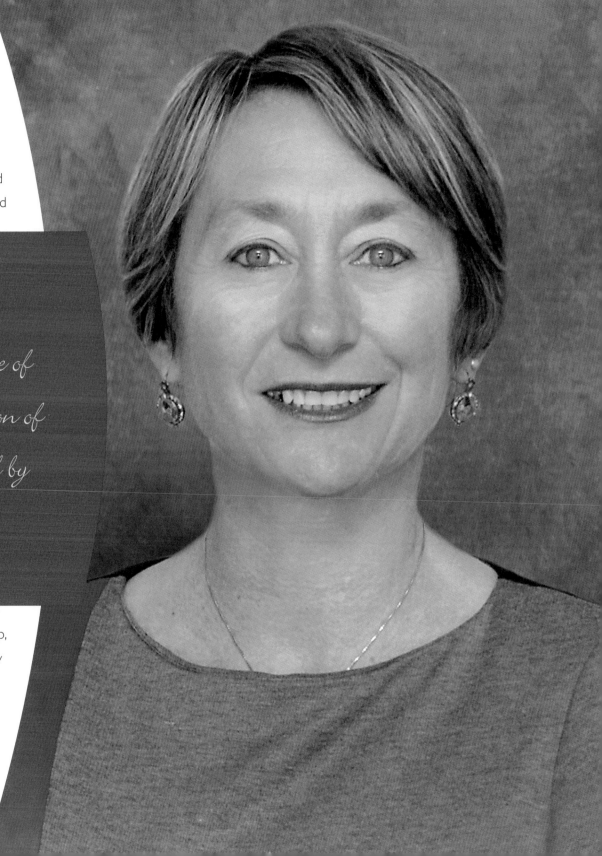

Our vision is, "Through creative leveraging of technology, UC College of Nursing will lead the transformation of health care in partnership informed by the people we serve."

men who create and live our legacy every day. Their leadership, innovation and commitment to care are what tell the real story of our history. Today our mantra is "UC Nurses. We See Leaders." It is clear to me that we have a legacy of leaders dating back to our roots in 1889.

Dean Greer Glazer, RN, CNP, PhD, FAAN

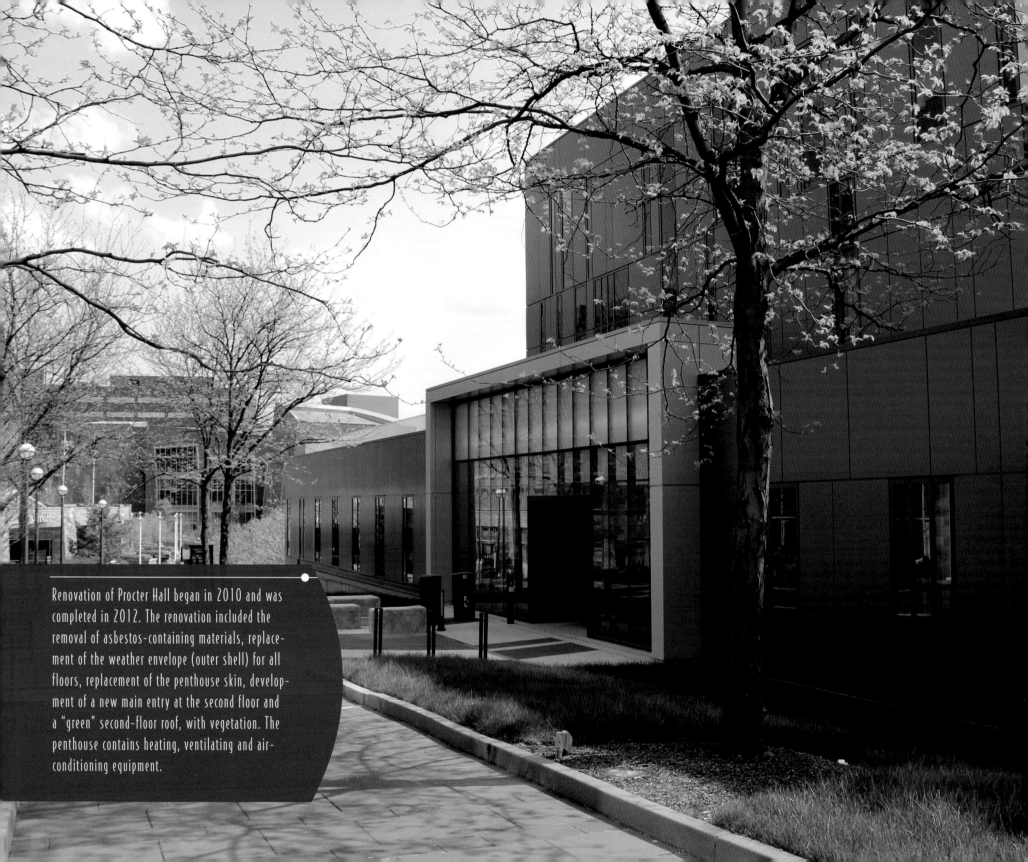

Renovation of Procter Hall began in 2010 and was completed in 2012. The renovation included the removal of asbestos-containing materials, replacement of the weather envelope (outer shell) for all floors, replacement of the penthouse skin, development of a new main entry at the second floor and a "green" second-floor roof, with vegetation. The penthouse contains heating, ventilating and air-conditioning equipment.

These leaders include the first nurses to graduate with a Bachelor of Science in Nursing degree. They include the first master's-prepared nurses. They include educators who overcame geographic boundaries with technology before computers were a staple in the average home. They include early nurse researchers. They include nurse administrators who have changed nursing practice. And they include nurses who have transformed countless individuals' and families' lives because of their never-ending commitment to quality care.

Today, we continue to innovate in the areas of education, research and practice. Our vision is "Through creative leveraging of technology, UC College of Nursing will lead the transformation of health care in partnership informed by the people we serve." Our faculty, staff, students and alumni continue to demonstrate the strong leadership and partnership prioritized so highly by our institution and so critical in achieving our vision.

In closing, this book is not the full or final story of University of Cincinnati College of Nursing. It's the story of our roots and our foundation. It's the story of how we created an infrastructure of evolution and innovation in nursing education. It's the story of our beginning—upon which we are building our future.

I hope that you will join me in celebrating our first 125 years and in shaping the next. It takes all of us working together to transform

health care. In the late 1800s, our founders and supporters believed in a vision and mission to improve health care. I personally hope that you'll do the same for the patients' lives that will be touched by UC nurses educated during the next 125 years.

Cheers to a healthy future!

Greer Glazer

Greer Glazer, RN, CNP, PhD, FAAN
Dean, University of Cincinnati College of Nursing
Schmidlapp Professor of Nursing
Associate Vice President for Health Affairs

UNIVERSITY OF
Cincinnati
COLLEGE OF
Nursing

CREATING A SCHOOL 1889–1899

Chapter One

1

In the late 1880s, the state of health care in Cincinnati was a paradox. On the one hand, the city, the densest in the United States with a population of approximately 300,000 people, was blessed with five hospitals—thanks to medical pioneers like Drs. Daniel Drake and Christian Holmes. One of the five was the very first Jewish Hospital in the United States, formed in response to the cholera epidemic of the 1840s.

On the other hand, however, working side by side with those doctors were untrained nurses and even family members, helping to care for the patients. As a result, patient care and outcomes were inconsistent. In fact, some sources blame the spread of the cholera on those untrained nurses as they went from house to house, comforting the ill and assisting their families.

Although Cincinnati had five hospitals, conditions in the hospitals were not very sanitary. In fact, the wealthy were usually treated at home until their care demanded care more sophisticated or technical than home visits could accomplish. Those people of the middle class held off going until they were near death, thus the hospitals were associated with dying. And the diseases that were being treated there were often incurable: tuberculosis, syphilis, infantile blindness from maternal gonorrhea—in addition to the aforementioned cholera epidemics.

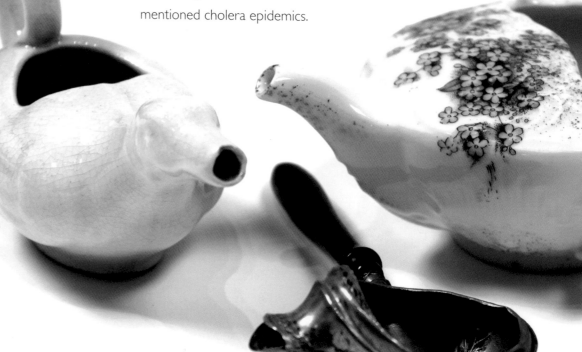

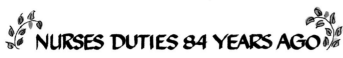

NURSES DUTIES 84 YEARS AGO

The following job description was given to floor nurses by a hospital in 1887:

In addition to caring for your 50 patients, each nurse will follow these regulations:

Daily sweep and mop the floors of your ward, dust the patients furniture and window sills. Maintain an even temperature in your ward by bringing in a scuttle of coal for the day's business. Light is important to observe the patient's condition. Therefore, each day fill kerosene lamps, clean chimneys and trim wicks. Wash the windows once a week. The nurse's notes are important in aiding the phsician's work. Make your pens carefully; you may whittle nibs to your individual taste. Each nurse on day duty will report every day at 7 a.m. and leave at 8 p.m. except on the Sabbath on which day you will be off from 12 noon to 2 p.m. Graduate nurses in good standing with the director of nurses will be given an evening off each week for courting purposes or two evenings a week if you go regularly to church. Each nurse should lay aside from each pay day a goodly sum of her earnings for her benefits during her declining years so that she will not become a burden. For example, if you earn $30 a month you should set aside $15. Any nurse who smokes, uses liquor in any form, gets her hair done at a beauty shop, or frequents dance halls will give the director of nurses good reason to suspect her worth, intentions and integrity. The nurse who performs her labors and serves her patients and doctors without fault for five years will be given an increase of five cents a day providing there are no hospital debts outstanding.

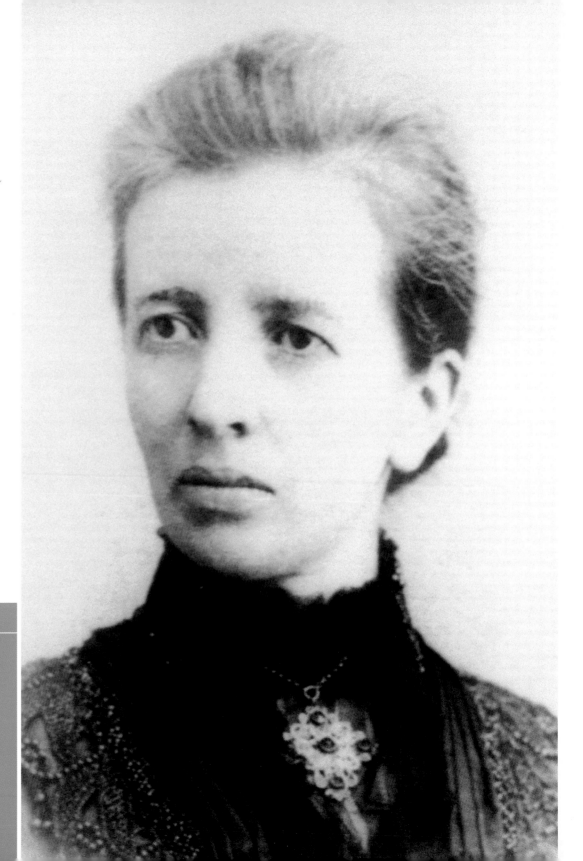

Left: Student nurses might have used baby feeders like these in the hospitals or in the homes. Baby feeders on loan to the Wedbush Nursing Legacy Centre from Dorothy Oechsler, founder and former director, Nursing Associate Degree Program, UC Blue Ash.
Top: Nurses' Duties of the Mid-19th Century.
Right: Superintendent Annie Murray, 1889–1893.

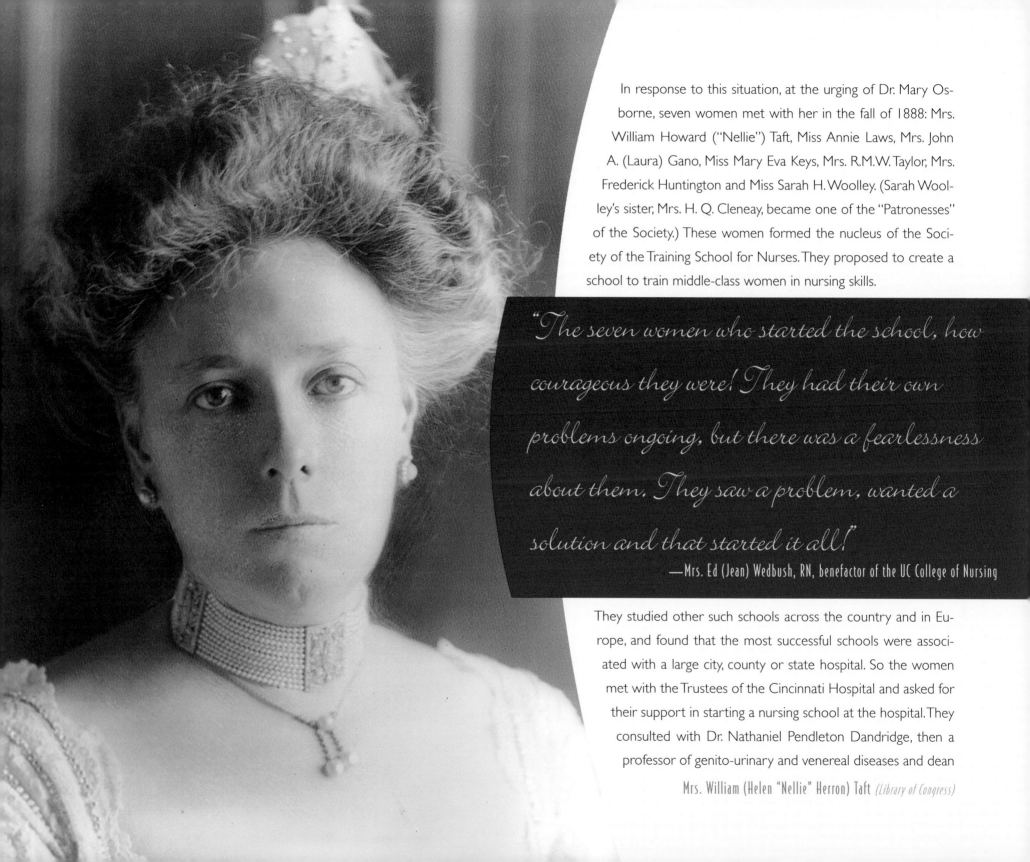

In response to this situation, at the urging of Dr. Mary Osborne, seven women met with her in the fall of 1888: Mrs. William Howard ("Nellie") Taft, Miss Annie Laws, Mrs. John A. (Laura) Gano, Miss Mary Eva Keys, Mrs. R.M.W. Taylor, Mrs. Frederick Huntington and Miss Sarah H. Woolley. (Sarah Woolley's sister, Mrs. H. Q. Cleneay, became one of the "Patronesses" of the Society.) These women formed the nucleus of the Society of the Training School for Nurses. They proposed to create a school to train middle-class women in nursing skills.

"The seven women who started the school, how courageous they were! They had their own problems ongoing, but there was a fearlessness about them. They saw a problem, wanted a solution and that started it all."

—Mrs. Ed (Jean) Wedbush, RN, benefactor of the UC College of Nursing

They studied other such schools across the country and in Europe, and found that the most successful schools were associated with a large city, county or state hospital. So the women met with the Trustees of the Cincinnati Hospital and asked for their support in starting a nursing school at the hospital. They consulted with Dr. Nathaniel Pendleton Dandridge, then a professor of genito-urinary and venereal diseases and dean

Mrs. William (Helen "Nellie" Herron) Taft *(Library of Congress)*

of the Miami Medical College. (It joined the University of Cincinnati in 1909, merging with the competing Medical College of Ohio.) Dr. Dandridge was very supportive of their cause. The Trustees of Cincinnati Hospital concurred, and—after adequate funds were raised—put the society and school in charge of the obstetrics ward (Ward Q) of the Cincinnati Hospital.

"The applicants were asked questions that today would send a human resources specialist screaming."

The model they chose to base their school on was the Bellevue Hospital School of Nursing in New York City, the first in the United States to be developed after the design of the Florence Nightingale School of Nursing, but the second training school for nurses after that of the New England Hospital for Women and Children. In 1880, only 15 such schools existed. By 1890, 35 nursing schools had been established; this number expanded to 432 by the turn of the century.

However, to create such a school would cost four thousand dollars. The society developed a brochure to describe their vision for the school and asked for donations. Two leading Cincinnatians were especially generous: Mrs. Bellamy (Maria Longworth Nichols) Storer and William A. Procter, son of William Procter, the co-founder of Procter & Gamble.

They determined their objectives to "first benefit patients by remedying defects of the old system of nursing by having a more carefully selected and competent class of nurses, to whom thorough training in all details relating to the well-being and comfort of patients be given. Second, to aid the physician."

The fundraising brochure described some of the goals of the Cincinnati Training School for Nurses as follows:

- "We require that a woman be sober, honest and truthful, without which there is no foundation on which to build.
- "We train her in the habits of punctuality, quietness, trustworthiness and personal neatness; we teach how to manage the concerns of a large ward or establishment.
- "We train her in dressing wounds and other injuries and in performing all those minor operations which nurses are called upon day and night to undertake.
- "We teach her how to manage helpless patients in regard to moving, changing, feeding, temperature and the prevention of bed sores.
- "She has to make and apply bandages, line splints for fractures and the like. She must know how to make beds with as little disturbance as possible to their inmates.
- "She is instructed how to wait operations, and as to the kind of aid the surgeon requires at her hands. She is taught cooking for the sick; the principles on which sick wards ought to be cleansed, aired and warmed; the management of convalescents, and how to observe sick and maimed patients, so as to give an intelligent and truthful account to the physician or surgeon is a much more difficult thing than is generally supposed.

Supporters of the Cincinnati Training School for Nurses

Many of these names include the most prominent Cincinnati families of the time and even today.

Managers

Miss Annie Laws
Mrs. John A. Gano
Mrs. F. G. Huntington
Mrs. J. D. Brannan
Mrs. R. M. W. Taylor
Mrs. Henry Stettinius
Mrs. John R. Holmes
Mrs. Herbert Jenney
Mrs. A. Hinkle
Mrs. Bellamy Storer
Miss Carson
Miss Eva Mary Keys
Miss Davis
Miss Sachs
Miss Woolley
Miss Neave
Mrs. L. C. Weir
Mrs. William A. Procter
Mrs. James M. Glenn
Mrs. Morris White
Mrs. Charles Anderson, Jr.
Mrs. Charles P. Taft
Mrs. William Ellis
Mrs. Cooper Procter

Patronesses

Mrs. Robert Burnet
Mrs. M. E. Ingalls

Mrs. A. S. Winslow
Mrs. I. J. Friedlander
Mrs. J. G. Schmidlapp
Mrs. Murat Halstead
Mrs. Lucien Wulsin
Mrs. John Henry
Mrs. Thomas Sherlock
Mrs. Rufus King, Jr.
Mrs. Telford Groesbeck
Mrs. Stewart Shillito
Mrs. R. R. Bowles
Mrs. Lewis VanAntwerp
Mrs. Aaron F. Perry
Mrs. Frederick Eckstein
Mrs. Frank J. Jones
Mrs. John Kilgour
Mrs. Louise N. Anderson
Mrs. Charles T. Dickson
Mrs. Frank Lawson
Mrs. James Espy
Mrs. Charles W. Short
Mrs. Lewis Seasongood
Mrs. W. W. Seely
Mrs. Elliott Pendleton, Jr.
Mrs. Albert H. Chatfield
Mrs. William J. Breed
Mrs. George K. Shoenberger
Mrs. James H. Laws
Mrs. Samuel B. Keys

Mrs. John A. Murphy
Mrs. John W. Herron
Mrs. Charles W. Woolley
Mrs. John H. Martin
Mrs. Harley T. Procter
Mrs. Frank Ellis
Mrs. Andrew Hickenlooper
Mrs. Herman Goepper
Mrs. Theodore Cook
Mrs. Harry Quinton Cleneay
Mrs. Frederick Eckstein, Jr.
Mrs. N. H. Davis
Mrs. Thomas P. Gaddis
Mrs. Joseph H. Crane
Mrs. Frank J. Patterson
Mrs. William McKinley, Jr.
Mrs. Ernst Lindsay
Mrs. James E. Campbell
Mrs. John B. Tytus
Mrs. William P. Orr
Mrs. L. O. Maddux
Mrs. George P. Wilshire
Mrs. George Davie
Mrs D. D. Bell
Mrs. J. S. Wayne
Mrs. Robert H. Shoemaker

Patrons

M. E. Ingalls

W. M. Ramsey
Alexander McDonald
Theodore Cook
William Hooper
Levi C. Goodale
William Woods
William H. Alms
Thomas Sherlock
James Espy
Julius Freiberg
Dr. David Judkins
Dr. John A. Murphy
Dr. P. S. Conner
Dr. Joseph Ransohoff
Hon. James E. Campbell
William A. Procter
Robert Mitchell
Robert B. Bowler
John A. Gano
Lowe Emerson
James Lowman
Leopold Feiss
John W. Herron
Robert Allison
W. H. Doane
Herbert Jenney
J. N. Kinney
F. H. Lawson
Adolph J. Seasongood

Hon. William McKinley, Jr.
Lewis Seasongood
J. T. Carew
A. J. Friedlander
John E. Bell
Frederick G. Huntington
J. D. Brannon
M. M. White
S. B. Keys
A. Caldwell Neave
J. F. Meader
Hon. William H. Taft
Peter Rudolph Neff
T. H. C. Allen

Executive Committee

A. Howard Hinkle
M. E. Ingalls
Stewart Shillito
J. G. Schmidlapp
H. T. Procter, Treasurer
L. C. Weir
I. J. Friedlander

●— "We do not seek to make 'medical women' but simple nurses acquainted with the principles which they are required constantly to apply at the bedside.

●— "For the future Superintendent is added a course of instruction in the administration of a hospital, including of course, the linen arrangements and what else is necessary for a matron to be conversant with.

●— "There are those who think that all of this is intuitive in women that they are born so, or at least, that it comes to them without training. To such we say, by all means send us as many such geniuses as you can, for we are sorely in need of them."

THE FIRST Class

Now that the school had funding and support, the next step was to hire a superintendent. From many applicants, Miss Annie Murray, a graduate of the Royal Infirmary of Edinburgh, Scotland, was hired. Soon after her appointment, Murray was also named Matron of the Cincinnati Hospital and was charged with providing "leadership for nursing service." With this move she was now responsible for both training the new nurses in the school and overseeing the existing nursing care at the hospital.

On January 1, 1889, five students entered the two-year program: Ella Curley, Kathryn Major, Mathilda Pfeifer, Daisey Mae Labo and Josephine Kloth. The applicants were asked questions that today would send a human resources specialist screaming:

●— Are you a single woman?
●— Age?
●— Height?
●— Are you strong and healthy?
●— Are your sight and hearing perfect?
●— Have you any physical defects?
●— If a widow, have you children? How are they provided for?

Besides taking classes, the students also worked 12-hour shifts in the hospital, six days a week. They were allowed a half day off on Sunday to attend church (and were strongly encouraged to do so). Sunday afternoons were for social activities, preferably needlework or talking to the other students.

By April of the first year of the arrangement, the school requested additional areas of the hospital to be added to the students' clinical rotation to enhance their learning experience. This was done and by May four more wards were added. At the end of the first year, the hospital experienced a dramatic drop in deaths from septicemia following childbirth and a significant decrease in septic peritonitis. Cincinnati Hospital's chief of staff, Dr. C. G. Comegys, reported that the hospital had never been "so well kept" and was "clean in all respects." Four more wards were added, bringing the total to nine wards under the care of the Nursing School.

The students learned through a combination of lectures delivered by the hospital's medical staff and clinical—or "scientific"—work acquired by working with ward patients directly. The first-year pupil nurses, as they were called, took lessons, attended lectures and

In the next year, some second-year students were sent into the homes of the sick as "district nurses," a step toward including public

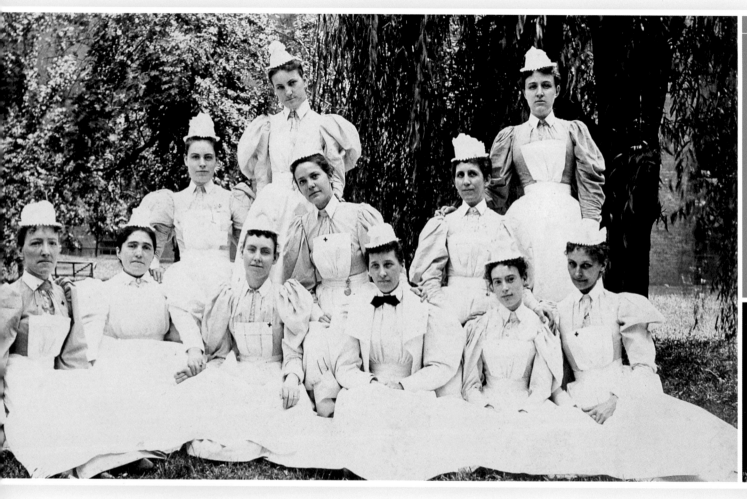

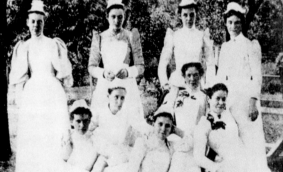

received practical experience in various aspects of nursing. These aspects included dressing blisters and sores; applying fomentations, poultices and leaches; administering enemas; cooking and serving "delicacies" for the sick; observing the state of secretions, intelligence, eruptions, pus and the effects of medicines.

health in the nursing program. The students might be sent to work in the hospital or in the homes of the rich or the poor.

Students were accepted on a rolling admission basis, so the class of 1891 had 11 graduating nurses: Mary Walters, Agnes Osborne, Bella Brace, Louise Lonsdale, Netta Donley and Mary Kimball (plus the original five). The school grew to 20 students in 1890 to 52 in 1891.

At the first commencement, January 1891, Society President Annie Laws told the graduates:

We feel that upon you depends the success or failure of our work. All the time, energy, thought, anxiety and money poured into this work would avail nothing if it did not produce as its result, earnest, faithful, conscientious, skilled nurses. As the pioneer class of the school, much has devolved upon you that may perhaps be spared other classes. We have watched your career during the past two years with an anxiety and an interest that can never be surpassed, if

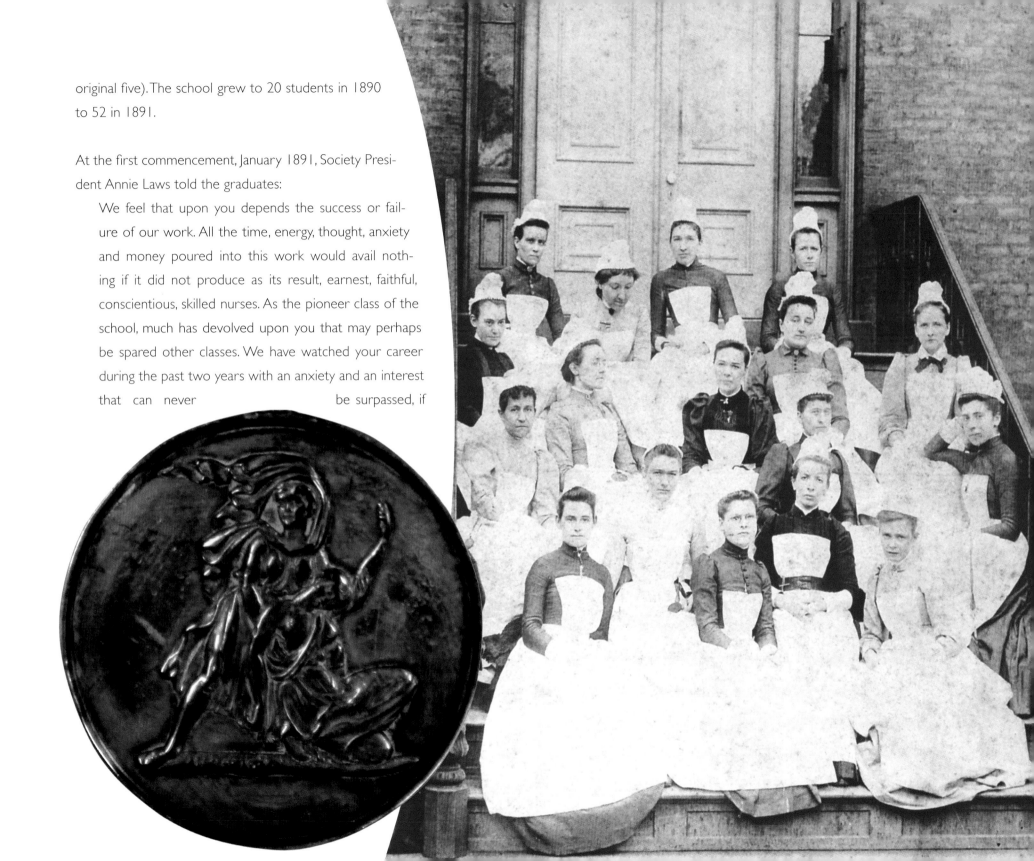

equaled, in the future. We have found you earnest and faithful, devoted to your work, ready in emergencies to do whatever might be required, and loyal always to the best interests of the school. Judging by the past, we feel that we can safely trust the reputation of the school in your hands. Hoping that while you are, in one sense, severing your connection with the school, in another, you will feel that you are always a part of it, and that you may always find in it whatever you may need in the future in the way of friendly counsel or aid, we wish you every success in your work, and believe that the Cincinnati Training School for Nurses will always have reason to be proud of its first class of graduates.

At this time, as Florence Nightingale, the "mother of modern nursing" fought for cleaner hospitals and sanitary conditions in Europe, in the 1890s schools of nursing began to spring up around the United States. However, the value of trained nurses to hospitals was not entirely altruistic: nursing students could provide a great deal of service to hospitals for little or no pay. Cincinnati Hospital, which had formerly been known as the public hospital for the poor or indigent, began to advertise its services to people of means, highlighting their trained nurses as one of the advantages of seeking care at Cincinnati Hospital.

At this point, the Cincinnati Training School for Nurses was funded entirely by donations, so each year meant another

round of fundraising was necessary. The American Medical Association was advocating that the medical profession (i.e., physicians) should fund and thereby control the nursing schools. Besides a funding question, this was also clearly a question of ego and control: the medical staff often stressed the nurse's role as "handmaiden to the physician." There was also a growing trend to have nursing schools controlled by the hospitals.

Meanwhile, Murray's dual role of superintendent of the nursing school and matron of nursing was causing conflict. The nurses who were at the hospital bristled under Murray's strict rules and refused to follow them. Murray had come directly to Cincinnati from a position as assistant matron at Philadelphia's Old Blockley. She was described as being a genteel lady with refined tastes and cultivated manners, which would have been an additional affront to the untrained nurses who had been at the hospital before her arrival.

Amidst all these conflicting forces, the school continued to grow. In fact, 1893 saw the graduation of the very first man from the school—Louis Lester—followed by Oriss O. Ross in 1897. (Some bedside care was deemed unsuitable for women.) As nursing became known as a "woman's profession," however, the numbers of men declined, and another male graduate was not seen again until 1976.

The struggle between the different entities came to a head over a charity ball held on January 21, 1892, to benefit the Training School for

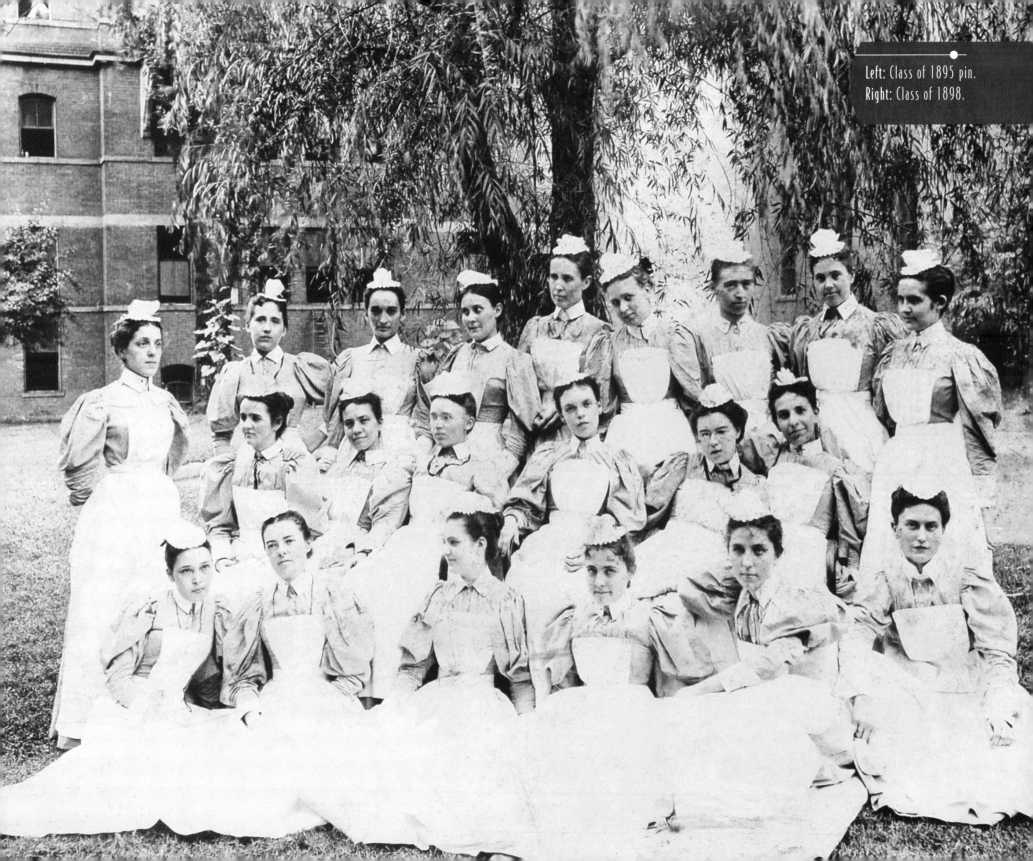

Nurses. The goal for the ball was to raise $10,000. However, E. W. Scripps, publisher of the *Cincinnati Post* started a smear campaign against the school in general and Annie Murray in particular. Scripps felt that women were happiest when left un-educated and "infirm" at home and that men should be in charge. The *Post* reported that the charity ball was a drunken affair, which made it difficult for the school to raise the needed funds.

Finally in 1893 the Society for the Training School for Nurses ad-mitted defeat in trying to maintain a nursing school independent of the hospital and withdrew its association from Cincinnati Hospital.

Then-U.S. Sixth Circuit Judge William Howard Taft spoke at the commencement exercises for the final graduation of the Training School for Nurses in January 1893. He expressed his pride at their accomplishments and his concern for the future. Thirty years later, another director of the School of Nursing, Laura R. Logan, said of the Society of the Training School for Nurses:

> The work of this group of Cincinnati women can hardly be overestimated. Not ony did they set a standard for nursing schools, which was rapidly taken up by other groups in the city, once the medical profession and the public had come to know the value of skilled nursing, but they also brought their work to the public by establishing a Directory for Nurses in September 1891. They also introduced trained nursing care into the Home for the Friendless, and the Soldiers' Homes at Dayton, Ohio, and Marion, Indiana. In the same year, they began the work of Visiting Nursing.

The hospital trustees then established their own school of nursing under their management and direction. They named Olive Fisher superintendent. Fisher had been Murray's second in command and was a graduate of Blockley Hospital in Philadelphia.

In 1894, with the new hospital school thriving, the trustees asked the city to provide a new home away from the hospital proper but still on the hospital grounds. Up until this point, nurses slept in the wards near their patients. In the preceding winter, several nurses had become ill, probably as a result of the long working hours and exacerbated by staying in small, unventilated rooms so close to the patients. Although the day shift nurses had been moved to independent apartments in 1890, the night nurses were not moved until 1892.

The hospital itself was also showing signs of wear. The hospital, lo-cated near the canal at 12th and Elm, was also susceptible to water-borne diseases and mosquitos. In the census of 1896 the Cincin-nati Hospital held 407 patients, over capacity, especially in facilities for contagious diseases. Dr. Christian Holmes felt that the hospital would gain advantages from being located close to the university.

At the end of the 19th century, the nurses were training at Cincinnati Hospital at Cincinnati Hospital Training School for Nurses. The pro-gram had been expanded to a three-year diploma program, consist-ing of an apprenticeship format learning from nursing staff at patients' bedsides and through classroom lectures in organized courses.

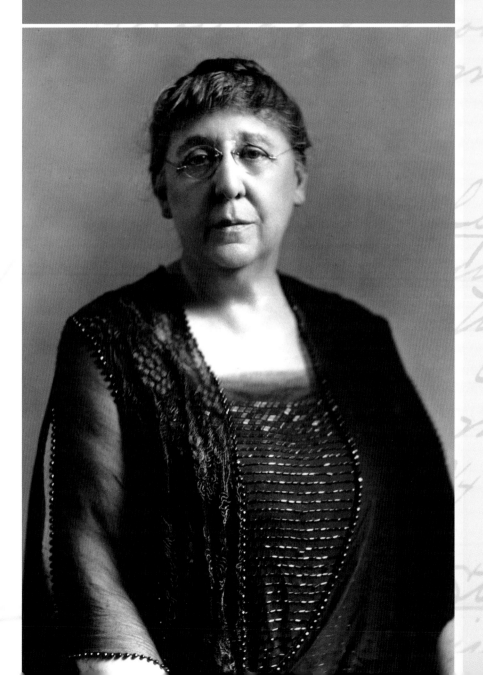

Bottom: Miss Annie Laws, the first manager of the Society of the Training School for Nurses.

Right (screen): Annie Murray kept a painstakingly detailed, hand-written book, which the next few superintendents kept up, of all the nurses enrolled in the school. She updated each record with the nurse's graduation date, grade and—where appropriate—marriage or death.

1889 Seven women started the Cincinnati Training School for Nurses as a small private school on January 1, 1889. Those seven founders were Mrs. John A. Gano, Mrs. Frederick G. Huntington, Miss Mary Eva Keys, Miss Annie Laws, Mrs R. M. W. Taylor, Miss Sarah H. Woolley and Mrs. William ("Nellie") Howard Taft. They first met in the office of Dr. Mary Osborne (minus Mrs. Taft).

1891 The first class graduated 11 students. Students back then were admitted on a rolling basis, so each "class" photo shows more students even though not all were ready to graduate.

1893 The first male graduated: Louis Lester. Back then, bedside care was not considered appropriate for young ladies. Nursing had not yet been completely defined as a "woman's profession."

1893 The school became the Cincinnati Hospital Training School for Nurses under control of the hospital and funded by the city of Cincinnati.

1894 The Alumni Association formed.

1897 The second male graduated: Oriss O. Ross.

IMPROVING PUBLIC HEALTH 1900–1909
Chapter Two

2

As the 20th century opened, the Cincinnati Hospital trustees were working to establish a nursing school under the auspices of the hospital. The new superintendent chosen was Olive Fisher, Annie Murray's former assistant. Under Fisher's watchful eye, the new Cincinnati Hospital Training School for Nurses grew from a two-year to a three-year diploma program, which was a trend in nursing schools at the time.

However, not everyone agreed on what that third year should be used for. Isabel Hampton Robb, superintendent of the Johns Hopkins School for Nursing and founder of the American Society of Superintendents of Training Schools for Nurses of the United States and Canada, favored the third year's focus being on education for the student. Most of the schools, however, which at that time were typically affiliated with hospitals, preferred having the students spend their third year getting practice on the floors of the hospital. It was no surprise that the hospitals supported

the solution that provided them with inexpensive labor. Student nurses fulfilled a great need in hospitals that were so overcrowded that in some cases patients were placed on the floor for lack of beds.

In such overcrowded conditions, sanitation was difficult. This was a time that many changes were being made to Cincinnati's city infrastructure. With increasing population after the Civil War, houses and businesses had been built but the sewer system had not kept up with the growth. By 1870, only 671 houses had been connected to city sewers. The others discharged their waste directly into the Mill Creek or Miami & Erie Canal. Homes farther away from downtown dumped their waste into creeks that then emptied directly into the Ohio River. The sewage problem was not quickly or easily solved.

Meanwhile, transportation changes offered new dangers on the streets of Cincinnati. Horse-drawn street cars had begun operating in 1859 and were the preferred mode of transportation. However, as popular as the street cars were, Cincinnatians were finding it difficult to make the trip up the many hills. The hills were too steep for the horses to pull full loads up, so "inclined planes"—inclines, for short—were constructed.

The Mount Auburn incline, opening in spring 1872, was the first to be finished. It ran from Main Street up to Jackson Hill. It was followed

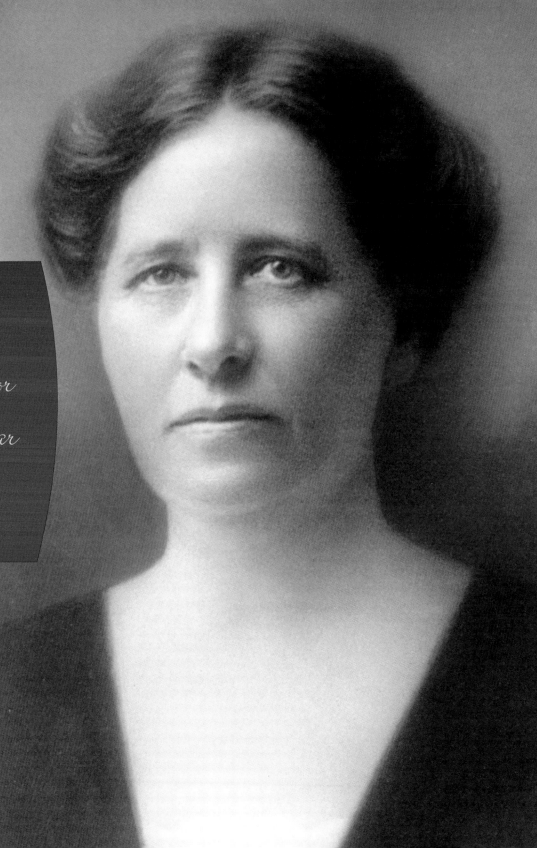

Under Fisher's watchful eye, the new Cincinnati Hospital Training School for Nurses grew from a two-year to a three-year diploma program.

quickly by four more inclines: the Clifton (or Bellevue), the Fairview, the Mount Adams and Price Hill. A terrible accident occurred on the Mount Auburn incline on Oct. 15, 1889, when the car broke free of its cable and raced down the incline, crashing at the bottom. Three passengers died at the scene. Three others were rushed to Cincinnati Hospital, where nurses from the school cared for them along with physicians, but to no avail. Their injuries were too great and they later died. The other passenger was injured

Left: 1903 class pin.
Right: Superintendent Olive Fisher, 1893–1911.

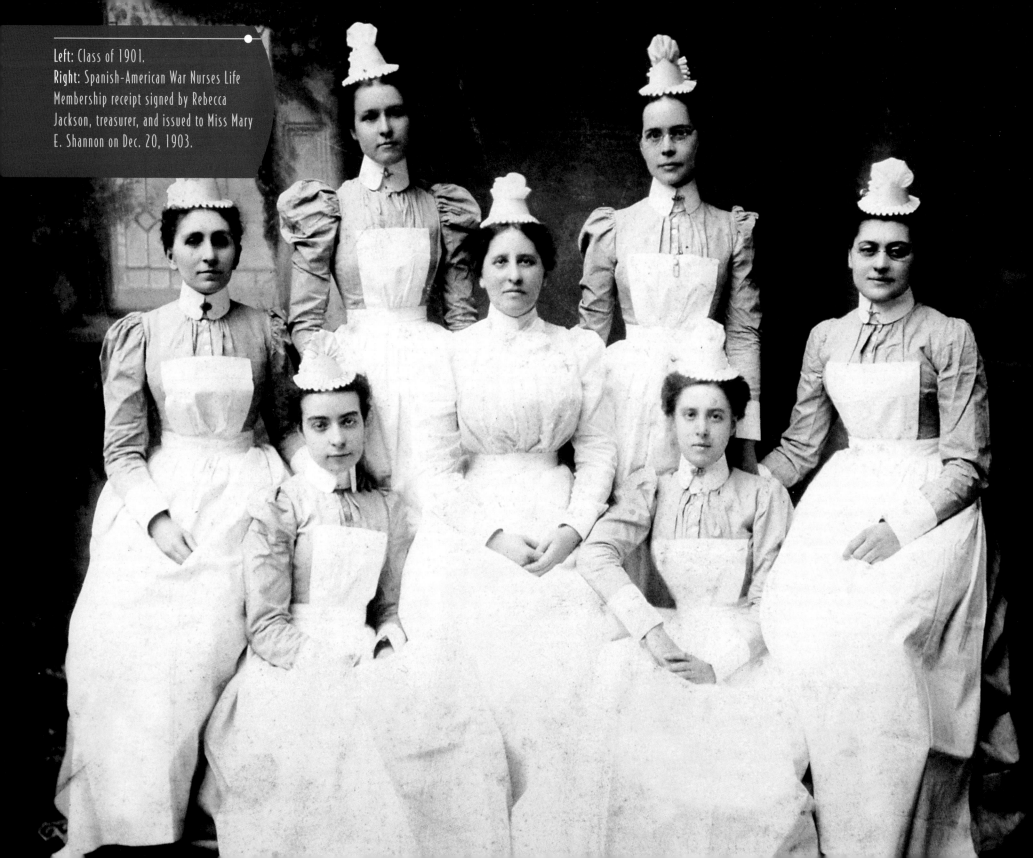

but recovered. The incline was shut down and remodeled. Eventually, this incline outlasted all the others, finally being shut down in 1948.

to Ohio Avenue. The Clifton (also known as the Bellevue Incline) ran from 1876 to 1926.

Spanish-American War Nurses.

LIFE MEMBERSHIP.

ISSUED _December 26th_ 190 3

MISS _Mary E. Shannon_ TO

AS A RECEIPT FOR

$10.00 LIFE MEMBERSHIP FEE.

Rebecca Jackson

TREASURER.

The Fairview Incline ran from 1892 to 1923. The Fairview was unique in that it was originally built for streetcars, but ended up being used by passengers only—no horses. The other inclines (save Price Hill's) were built for passengers and ended up being converted for street car use. The Fairview Incline ran from McMicken Avenue to Fairview Avenue. Clifton's incline from Elm and McMicken streets

Soon thereafter cable cars made their appearance, climbing the less steep—but still imposing—Gilbert Avenue from downtown to Peebles Corner. Cincinnati legend has it that Mr. Peebles, of the Joseph R. Peebles' Sons Co. grocery store, paid the cable car conductors a little on the side to shout out "Peebles Corner!" as they crested the hill and to make it a stop. Prior to this, the intersection of Gilbert and McMil-

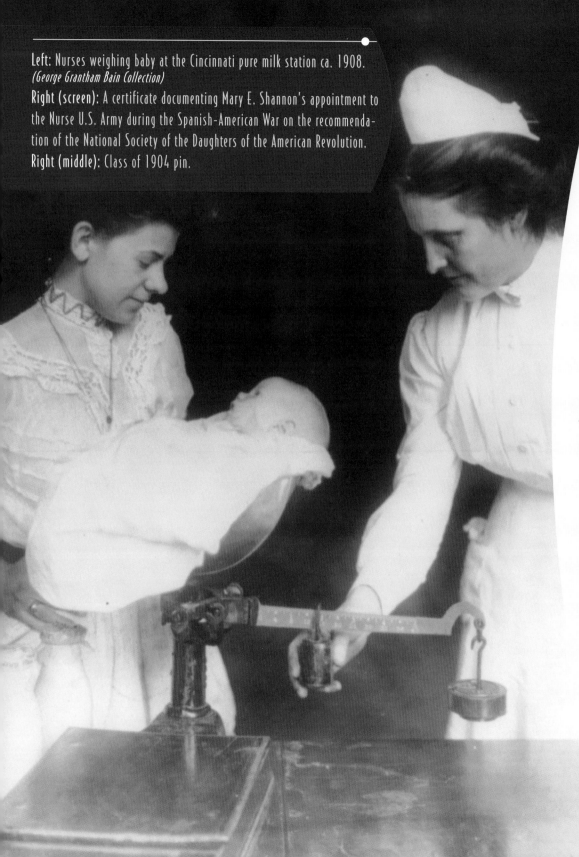

lan had been known as Kay's Corner—for the Kay grocery shop on the other corner.

Changes were occurring in the health scene in Cincinnati, as well. Christian R. Holmes, a native of Denmark, had earned his medical doctor's diploma from the Cincinnati College of Medicine and Surgery at the age of 29. At first, he entered private practice and made quite a name for himself through his widely read publications. Three years after his graduation, he was elected president of the local Medical Society. He married Bettie Fleischmann (23 years his junior) in 1892, which made him brother-in-law to Mayor Julius Fleischmann (the youngest mayor of Cincinnati to this day).

In 1900 Dr. Holmes became a trustee of Cincinnati Hospital, which at that point was in horrible shape with unsanitary conditions and lacking equipment. Dr. Holmes' dream was to have a modern hospital with a better medical school and better education, based on the Johns Hopkins model where surgeons would be trained to serve the community. Dr. Holmes battled different mayors and worked to raise money and support from the public. He spent the entire first decade of the 20th century working toward his dream of a clean, modern teaching hospital.

Meanwhile, the medical colleges were not in much better shape than the hospitals that hosted them. The College of Medicine and Surgery closed in 1902, replaced in function by the Miami Medical College and the Medical College of Ohio (founded by Dr. Daniel Drake). After the College of Medicine and Surgery closed, the Miami and Ohio medical colleges remained open but foundering and contentious. Nevertheless, the two united in 1906 as the Ohio-Miami Medical College. Within three years it joined the University of Cincinnati as the Ohio-Miami Medical Department.

The hospital at this time was at the corner of 12th and Elm streets, adjacent to the Miami & Erie Canal. Patients often had to be draped with netting to fend off offensive flies and mosquitos. (In 1900, Walter Reed had proven that infected mosquito bites caused yellow fever.) The cholera epidemics of the mid-19th century had been blamed partially on the canal. And with all the raw sewage being dumped into it, the smell could not have been pleasant—especially in the summer months.

Dr. Holmes desperately wanted a new physical hospital facility and began "pounding the pavement" for money. He raised $7,500 from the general population, in an early version of "crowd-sourcing." Mrs. Mary ("Guppy" to her friends) Emery donated a quarter of a million dollars and challenged her peers to step up to the plate. Several Cincinnatians, whose names are still familiar today, rose to her challenge. Of special note are Mrs. Charles Fleischmann (Dr. Holmes' sister-in-law), William Cooper Procter (the grandson of Procter & Gamble co-founder William Procter) and Charles P. and Anna Taft— all of whom gave $50,000. Mrs. Bettie (Fleischmann) Holmes even gave $10,000 of her own money.

In 1904, the Ohio State Nurses' Association met in the library of the City Hospital on January 27 and 28. Annie Laws, one of the founders of the Society of the Training School for Nurses, delivered the "Ad-

dress of Welcome" in her capacity of president of the International Kindergarten Union. Other dignitaries in the medical field addressed the group, followed by the business meeting of the Graduate Nurses' Association. One of those in attendance was Olive Fisher, who was vice president at the time of the Graduate Nurses' Association. Following the meeting, a bill requiring that nurses be registered was prepared for submission to the state legislature.

With Florence Nightingale's heroic efforts in Europe, the end of the 19th century had certainly seen the value of sanitary conditions. For the first time, instruments were sanitized. The beginning of the 20th century also saw a move from home-taught nursing to hospital-based nursing education. With an influx of immigrants, nurses now began visiting people in their homes, whether they were houses, apartments or tenements.

An awakening was taking place in the profession of nursing in the United States in the first decade of the 20th century. The Army Nurse Corps was founded in 1901, which— with Jane Delano as superintendent—recruited nurses for the Red Cross Nurse Reserves and helped supply more than 20,000 nurses to serve in World War I. The Army Nurse Corps was followed by the development of the Navy Nurse Corps in 1907.

In 1905, the *American Journal of Nursing* was published for the first time with Mary E. P. Davis as managing editor. Davis espoused the idea of nurses as more than just "cheap labor."

And in 1908, Martha Minerva Franklin organized the National Association of Colored Graduate Nurses—a year *before* the National Association for the Advancement of Colored People (NAACP) was founded. Franklin had been the only African-American graduate of the "Woman's Hospital Training School" in Philadelphia, which had been founded in 1861.

So as the decade came to a close, nurses were focused on many issues on many fronts—equality, sanitation, respect, medicine—but the bottom line was still care for the patient.

Also as the decade came to a close, an elderly Florence Nightingale approached her 90th birthday. In 1893, Lystra Gretter, an instructor at Detroit's Harper Hospital, had written a variation of the physician's Hippocratic Oath for their graduating nurses. It has forever since been known as the Nightingale Pledge:

> I solemnly pledge myself before God and in the presence of this assembly, to pass my life in purity and to practice my profession faithfully. I will abstain from whatever is deleterious and mischievous, and will not take or knowingly administer any harmful drug. I will do all in my power to maintain and elevate the standard of my profession, and will hold in confidence all personal matters committed to my keeping and all family affairs coming to my knowledge in the practice of my calling. With loyalty will I endeavor to aid the physician in his work, and devote myself to the welfare of those committed to my care.

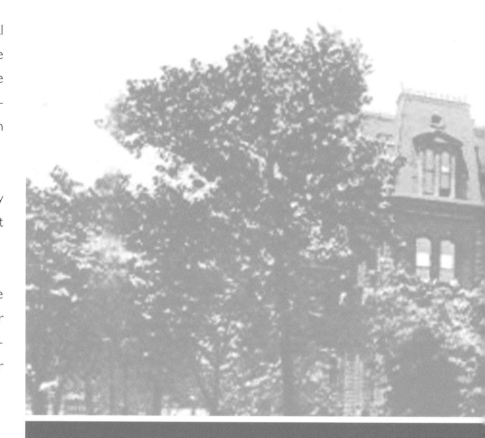

Left: Class of 1906 pin.
Right: Cincinnati Hospital.

1901–1909

1903 ● The three-year program was instituted.

1904 ● Alumni from 26 nursing schools in Ohio met at Cincinnati Hospital to form a state association of nurses. Those attending from Cincinnati became the nucleus of District 8 of the Ohio Nurses' Association.

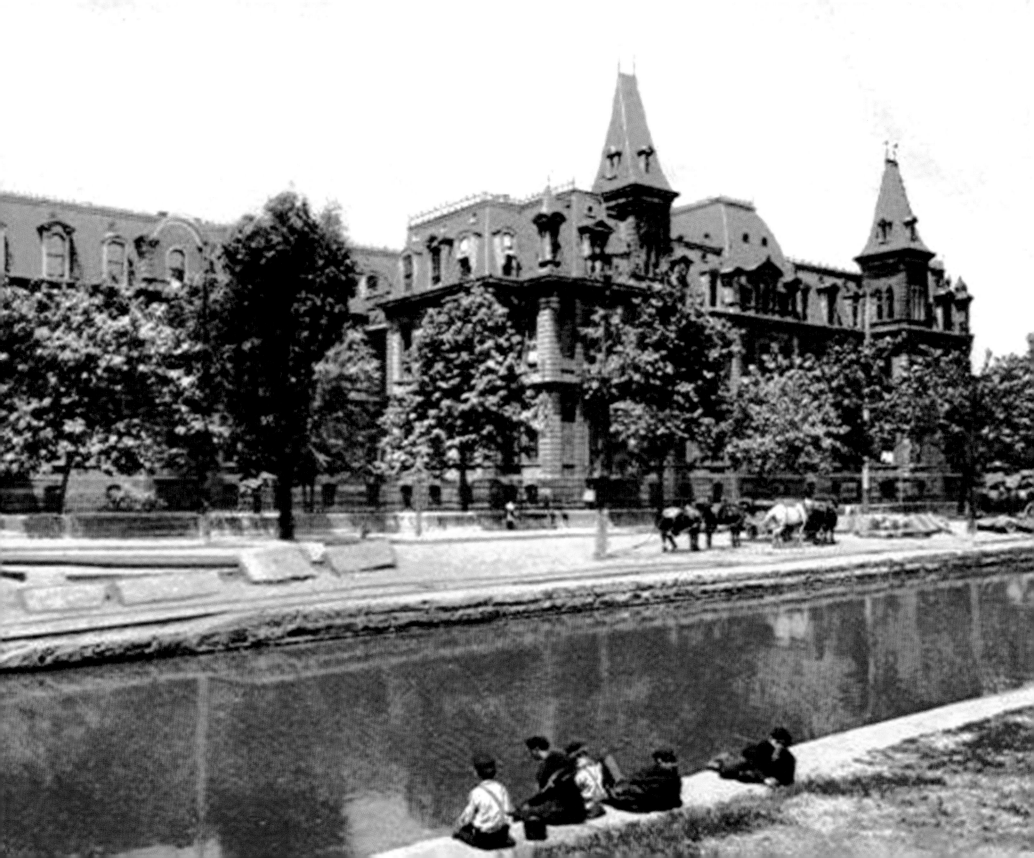

LEARNING NEW WAYS 1910–1919

Chapter Three

Sadly, the decade opened with the death of nursing pioneer Florence Nightingale, at the age of 90. Clearly, however, her voice would never be silenced. She had inspired nurses around the world and had established a connection between health and sanitation. Equally important, her voice had rung out on behalf of equality, human rights and patient care and well-being.

In the *Nurse and Hospital Review* of 1911, Lewellys F. Barker, MD, professor of medicine at Johns Hopkins University and Physician-in-Chief to Johns Hopkins Hospital, noted some changes in thinking that sound familiar to today's health practitioners:

One fact which has become ever clearer as medical knowledge has advanced concerns the nutrition of the child. Faulty feeding in infancy and early childhood may lead to such impoverishment of the tissues and such stunting of growth that the ill effects can never be recovered from in later life. A considerable proportion of the intellectual and moral in-

feriorities among our people is fairly attributable to imperfect nutrition at this early age. Fortunately the public is now being so thoroughly educated to the importance of breast feeding for infants and of liberal and suitable diet during the early years of life, by family physicians…and others on the care and feeding of children, that it is not necessary to dwell at length upon the subject. Plenty of good, simple food, including milk, meat, vegetables and fruit, with avoidance of condiments, coffee, tea and alcohol, is approved by all authorities.

Dr. Barker also noted some advice regarding the long-term benefits of exercise for children—and his concern that girls weren't being exposed to this same opportunity:

The boy who learns to tumble in a gymnasium, to stand the pain of boxing and fencing and wrestling and to keep his temper while engaging in these exercises will have subjected himself to a training which

Also according to the *Trained Nurse and Hospital Review*, the Graduated Nurses' Association of Cincinnati held a meeting in the library

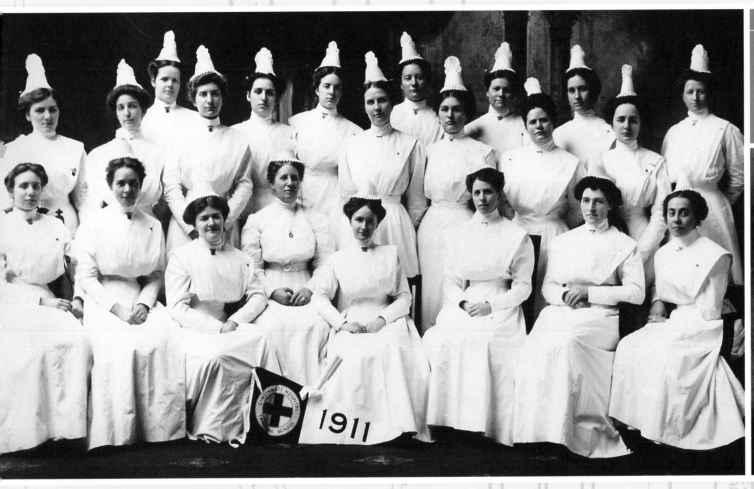

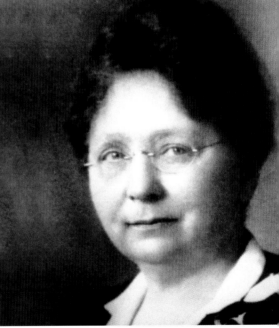

Left: A cord used for tying a baby's umbilical cord, 1911–1912.
Middle: Class of 1911.
Bottom: Director Katherine Ellison, 1911–1913.

cannot help but stand him in good stead later on in life. One reason why women are more prone in later life to nervousness than men may lie in the lessened opportunity which girls have for bodily and psychic hardening in the games which they play and the life which they lead as children.

of the Cincinnati Hospital on September 25. During the session Miss Olive Fisher, president of the association and superintendent of the nursing school, was presented with a silver tea urn. The presentation speech was made by Miss Mary Greenwood, superintendent of the Jewish Hospital nurses. The following subjects were discussed: Ida Hasselburg, "School Nursing"; Miss Bode, "Visiting Nurses"; Mary

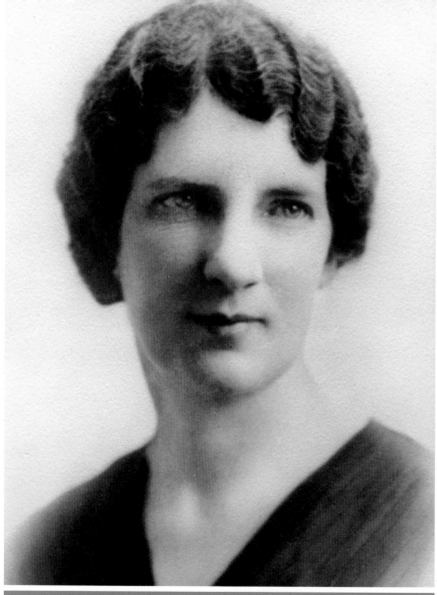

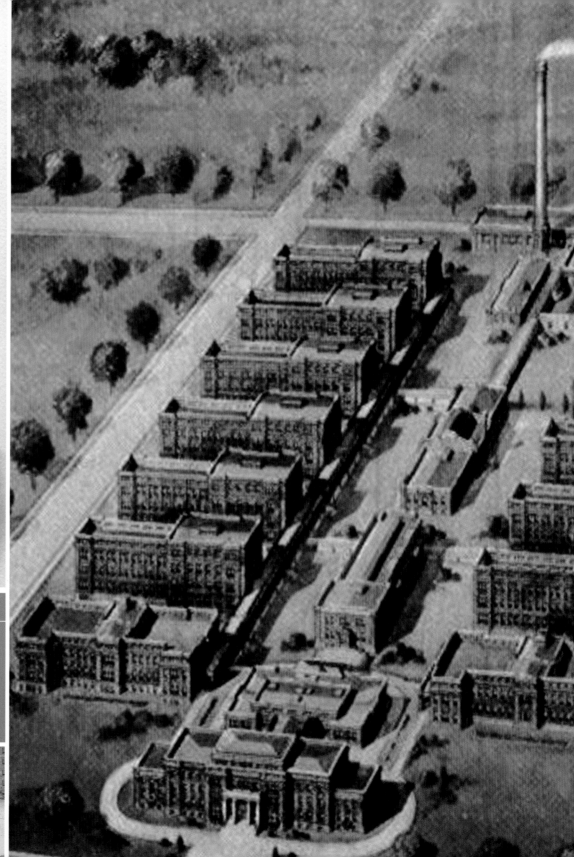

Top: Superintendent Marguerite Fagen, 1913–1914.
Bottom (left to right): Director Laura R. Logan, 1914–1915; 1918 Base Hospital #25.
Right: Bird's-eye view of the new General Hospital.

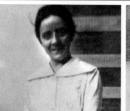

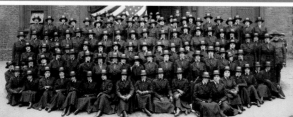

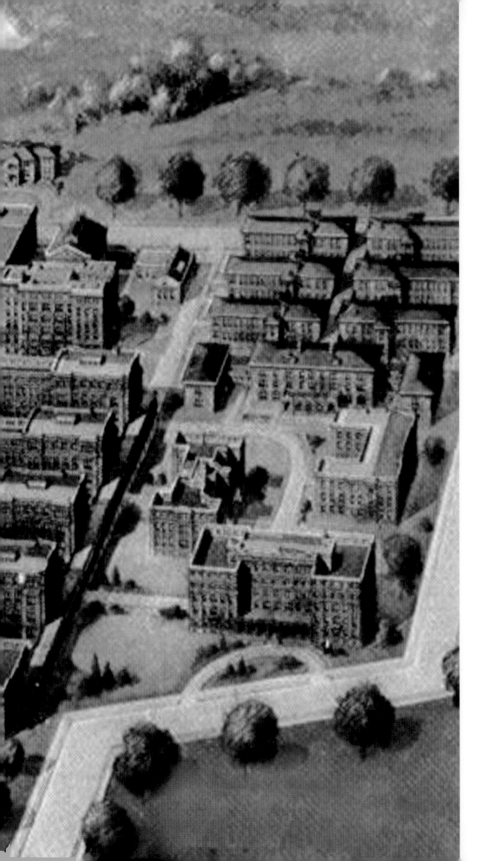

Emery, "Anti-Tuberculosis Nursing"; Ella Aurey, "Private Nursing," and Lena Mitchke, "Nursing of Blind Children." The subjects reflect the changes that had occurred in the beginning of the 20th century toward focusing on public health.

Cincinnati Hospital Training School Superintendent Olive Fisher had to retire after 18 years in 1911 because of failing health. She was replaced by alumna Katherine Ellison ('08), who became director of the school. Ellison held this position for two years until her classmate Marguerite Fagen became superintendent. Fagen held this position in 1913 and 1914.

This was the first such baccalaureate degree of its type in the United States. It was a major step in the evolution of nursing education.

On December 1, 1912, the *New York Times* announced, "The Finest Hospital in the World in Cincinnati." Dr. Christian Holmes became dean of the College of Medicine with Charles Dabney as president of the university. (He remained dean from 1914 until his death.) Finally, even working himself into frail health, his dream of a modern hospital came true. In January 1914 the new Cincinnati General Hospital, built by Samuel Hannaford & Sons, was completed and became part of the University of Cincinnati. Cities from around the country sent representatives to Cincinnati to study Dr. Holmes' hospital so they could mimic it.

Curriculum for Five-Year Program and Three-Year Diploma Program 1916-1917

Pre-Nursing Program

First Year

Chemistry 1, 2, 3, 4	10 hours
English	6 hours
Zoology 1, 2	10 hours
Hygiene	2 hours
Physical Education	2 periods per week
Total	**28 hours**

Second Year

Electives from the following group of subjects: psychology, economics, social science, political science, history, modern language, chemistry, philosophy, English, physics, mathematics, zoology and botany

	34 hours
Hygiene	2 hours
Physical Education	2 periods per week
Total	**36 hours**

Three-Year Program

First Term (Probation) 16-18 Weeks

THEORY		PRACTICE	
Elements of Nursing			
History and Ethics of Nursing	15 hours	Class & Practice	2 weeks
Personal and Hospital Hygiene	15 hours	Social Service and Admitting Pavilion	1 week
Clinical Techniques of Nursing (including Hospital and Household Economy)	15 hours	Medical Wards	4 weeks
Elementary Biology	15 hours	Surgical Wards	4 weeks
Pharmacy	30 hours	Children's Wards	4 weeks
Foods	6 hours	Operating Pavilion	1 week
Elements of Cooking	15 hours		

Second Term

THEORY		PRACTICE	
Chemistry	75 hours	6 hours relief on wards each Sunday only	
Anatomy & Physiology	75 hours		
Nutrition IV	60 hours		
Nursing	60 hours		

Third Term

THEORY		PRACTICE	
No classes during the summer		Diet Laboratory	1 month
Medical Wards	2 months		
Vacation	1 month		

Second Year, First Term

THEORY		PRACTICE	
Massage and Orthopedic Nursing	15 hours	Orthopedic Ward and Gymnasium	1 month
Pediatric Nursing	15 hours	Surgical Wards	2 months
Invalid Occupations	15 hours	Milk Laboratory	1 month

Second Term

THEORY		PRACTICE	
Bacteriology and Hygiene	75 hours	6 hours relief on wards each Sunday only	
Social Psychology	60 hours		
Sociology	60 hours		
Pharmacology and Therapeutics	30 hours		
Pathology	15 hours		

Third Term

THEORY		PRACTICE	
No classes during the summer		Gynecological Ward	1 month
		Operating Pavilion	1½ months
		Social Service and Admitting Pavilion	½ month
		Vacation	1 month

Third Year, First Term

THEORY		PRACTICE	
Nursing (Obstetricial- 20 hours, Communicable Diseases- 15 hours, Nervous and Mental- 10 hours, Eye, Ear, Nose, & Throat- 10 hours, Skin and Venereal- 5 hours)	15 hours	Contagious Wards	2 months
		Children's Wards	2 months

Second Term

THEORY		PRACTICE	
Nursing Methods	30 hours	Medical Nursing	1 month
Public Health Nursing	30 hours	Obstetrical Wards	2 months
Application of Preventive Medicine in Nursing	15 hours	Ear, Eye, Throat and Nose Wards	1 month

Third Term

THEORY		PRACTICE	
No classes in the summer, except those going into Public Health Nursing	60 hours	Psychopathic Wards	2 months
		Outpatient or Clinic	2 months
		Administration (Educational Course)	4 months
		Field Work (for those going into Public Health Nursing	4 months

Dr. Holmes' dream had come to fruition. The 850-bed Cincinnati General Hospital was now located in Avondale neighborhood, which at that time was the geographic center of the city. The layout of the hospital was based on the pavilion style that was popular at the time. Separate pavilions helped isolate patients by disease, and covered walkways or tunnels protected patients, visitors and caregivers as they traveled between buildings. In the event of an epidemic, an entire building could be easily quarantined, closed or—if need be—razed.

The nurses' home included classroom, living and recreation space. The name of the school was changed to the School of Nursing and Health of the Cincinnati General Hospital. In 1914, Laura R. Logan was offered the position of director of the newly named school. She accepted, upon condition that the school would be affiliated with a university. National support was growing for university-based nursing schools, as documented in a study by the National League of Nursing Education and the Goldmark Report and elsewhere.

In 1916, the School of Nursing and Health of Cincinnati General Hospital became a school in the College of Medicine in the University of Cincinnati. A three-year diploma course and a five-year degree course were offered. All students took three years of academic courses and clinical instruction offered at the School of Nursing and Health.

Students who wished to earn the Bachelor of Science in Nursing degree took a two-year pre-nursing course in liberal arts in the

Above: 1916 class pin.

McMicken College of Liberal Arts and Sciences before taking the three-year diploma sequence. This was the first such baccalaureate degree of its type in the United States. It was a major step in the evolution of nursing education.

Under Logan's leadership, the School of Nursing and Health experienced many other opportunities. Students in their third year could elect to have four weeks' experience within a specific area in the hospital, in private duty, or in public health. The curriculum was also redesigned so students learned theory related to a specific area of nursing and then had the opportunity to apply the theory in a related clinical area.

Another first in nursing—getting college credit for time spent in clinical duties—began at the University of Cincinnati School of Nursing and Health. This change emphasized the importance of hands-on practice based on academic theory learned in the classroom. As a result of these and other changes, Logan became in high demand as a speaker.

As a result of these changes, enrollments increased and the curriculum became more complex. With that came a need for greater record-keeping and a greater storage space. Mrs. Charles Schram donated the funds to enlarge the existing library, which was named the Solomon W. Levi Memorial Library in memory of her husband, one of the best-equipped nursing libraries in the country.

1914 A new nursing school and home were built as part of the new Cincinnati General Hospital. The name of the school was changed to the School of Nursing and Health of the Cincinnati General Hospital.

1915 Mrs. Charles H. Schram funded the creation of the "Solomon W. Levi Memorial Library."

1916 The School of Nursing and Health of the Cincinnati General Hospital became the School of Nursing and Health in the College of Medicine of the University of Cincinnati. The school offered both a three-year diploma program and a five-year baccalaureate degree. The school was the first in the United States to offer the baccalaureate degree. The educational program was reorganized to include collegiate courses in addition to the three-year hospital-based program. The result was a five-year combined baccalaureate program which granted the Bachelor of Science in Nursing degree.

1917 Senior students specialized by working four weeks in a specific clinical area in the hospital, in private duty, or in public health.

1918 The School of Nursing and Health became the first school in the United States to grant academic credit for clinical work.

1919 The School of Nursing and Health became the first school in the United States to graduate a student with a Bachelor of Science in Nursing *and* a diploma. The student, Parthinia K. Foster, had entered with advanced standing and was thus able to complete a five-year baccalaureate program in three years.

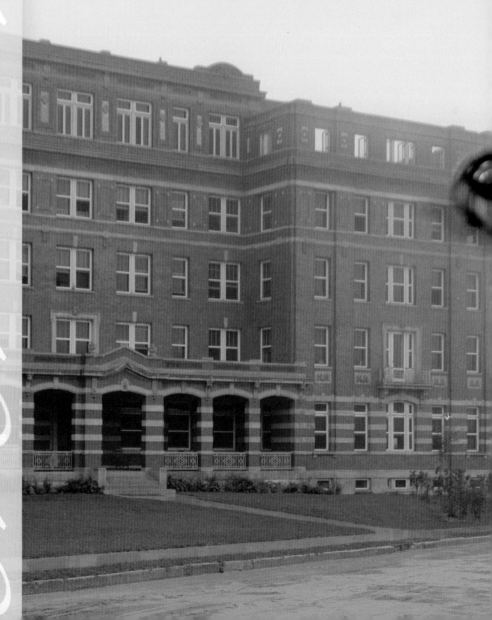

Left: Originally known as the General Hospital Nurses' Home, Logan Hall was designed in 1915 by Samuel Hannaford & Sons. It is listed on the National Historic Register and currently houses the Central Clinic for Behavioral Health and Forensic Services. *(Library of Congress)*
Right (left to right): Metal hypodermic syringe donated by Bertha Hellrung (Class of 1915); Part of the class of 1915.

Up until that time, the nursing students had worn their nurses' uniforms at graduation. However, now—in keeping with university tradition—the students from the School of Nursing and Health wore caps and gowns, and walked with students from the other colleges at the university at graduation. The first graduate of the new school and the first student in the United States to receive a Bachelor of Science degree and a diploma in nursing was Parthinia Katherine Foster, in 1919. (She was able to receive the degree so quickly because she had received advanced standing from courses already taken from the McMicken College of Liberal Arts and Sciences.)

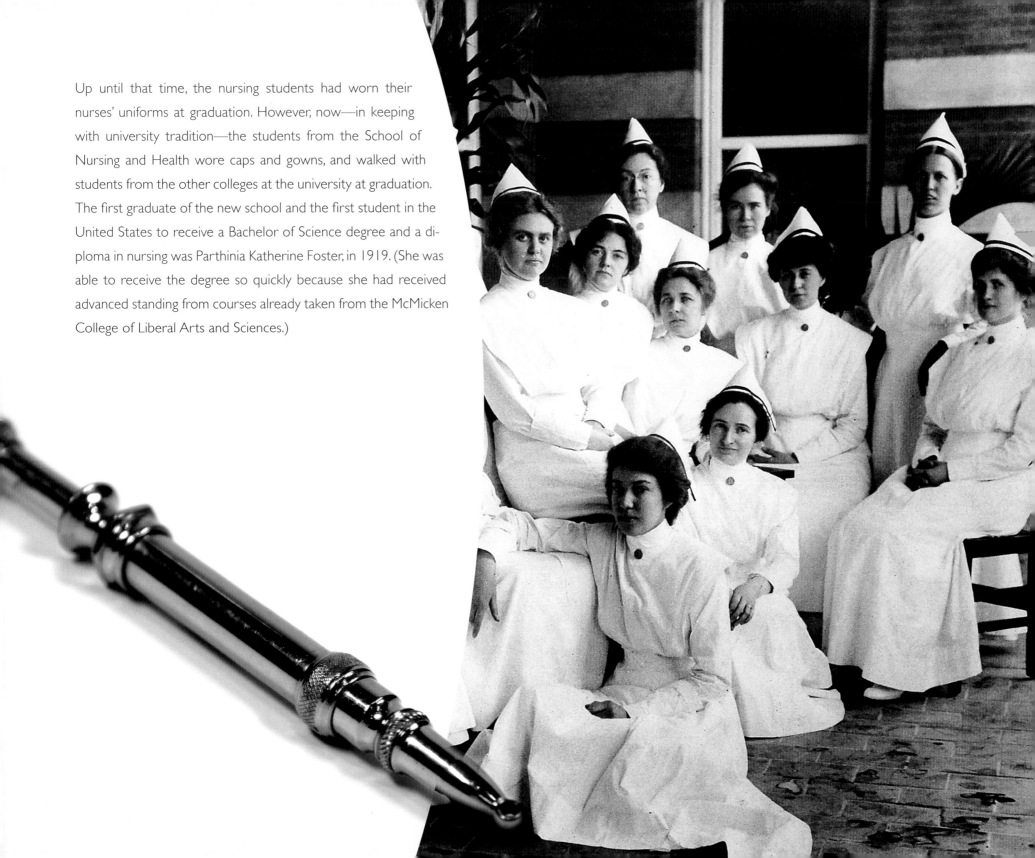

CHANGING TIMES 1920–1929

4

Once again, the decade opened with the loss of a pioneer. Dr. Christian Rasmus Holmes died on January 9, 1920, at the age of 62; some say he sacrificed his own health for the sake of the public's health and because of his dedication to fundraising. His widow continued his incredible efforts in his memory, building the private Holmes Hospital, planning the public Cincinnati General Hospital's kitchen and planning the nurses' building.

In November 1920, Laura R. Logan—then the director of the School of Nursing and Health of the College of Medicine—noted the contributions of the Society of the Training School for Nurses, that stalwart group of seven women who had met 31 years prior:

The work of this group of Cincinnati women can hardly be over-estimated. Not only did they set a standard for nursing schools, which was rapidly taken up by other groups in the city, once the medical profession and the public had come to know the value of skilled nursing, but they also brought their work to the public by establishing a Directory for Nurses in September 1891. They also introduced trained nursing care into the Home for the Friendless and the Soldiers'

Homes [in] Dayton, Ohio, and Marion, Indiana. In the same year they began the work of Visiting Nursing.

The National Soldiers' Home System had been established by President Abraham Lincoln during the Civil War. He recognized that many of the soldiers would not be able to return to their former lives and would need somewhere to go and some form of extended care. So on March 3, 1865, he signed the law establishing the National Asylum for Disabled Volunteer Soldiers (the law's name was changed in 1873 to the "National Home for Disabled Volunteer Soldiers," but the centers were known informally as "Soldiers' Homes"). Even after the Training School for Nurses was discontinued in Cincinnati, it continued to take care of the Soldiers' Homes in Dayton, Ohio, and Marion, Indiana, for a period of time.

The Soldiers' Home of Dayton, three miles west of Dayton, was a large facility, caring for 7,092 veterans (not all in-patients) in 1898. (Record-keeping was not consistent after this point.) John Lendrum Mitchell, the manager of the Milwaukee Soldiers' Home (the first such home) had recently contracted with nurses from the Wisconsin Training School for

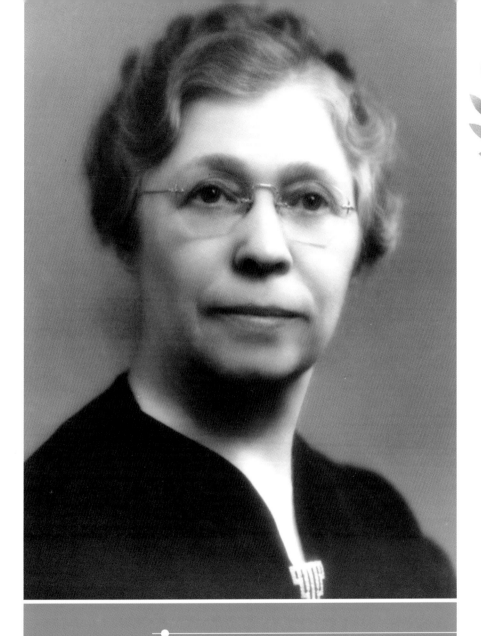

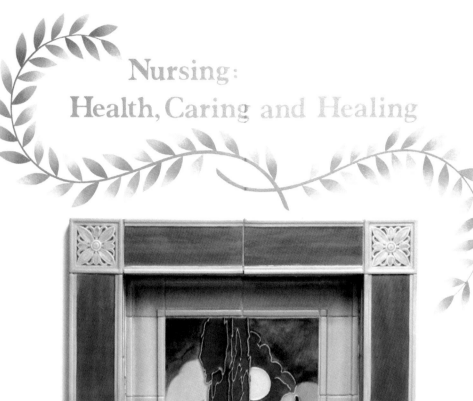

PRESENTED
BY THE
CLASS OF 1920

Top: Director Phoebe Kandel, 1925–1927.
Right: The Rookwood fountain was commissioned by the 1920 nursing class and placed in their Logan Hall residence. The 1992 nursing class restored and relocated the fountain to the present day College of Nursing, Procter Hall.

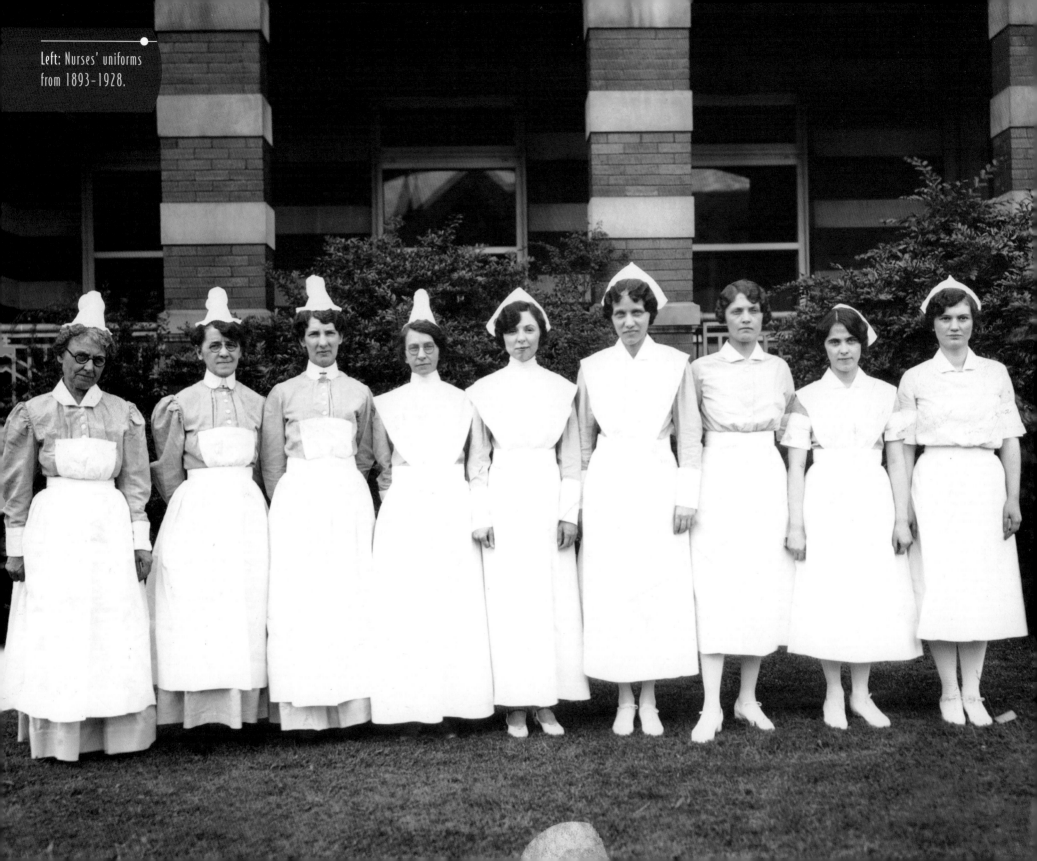

Female Nurses, bucking the previous trend for having men take care of the veterans:

the [nurses] training school in Cincinnati presumably. We have not as yet made any arrangements but I have no doubt

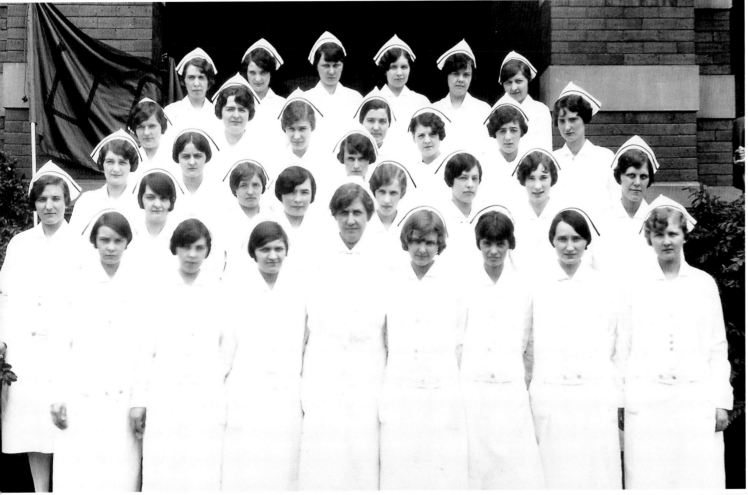

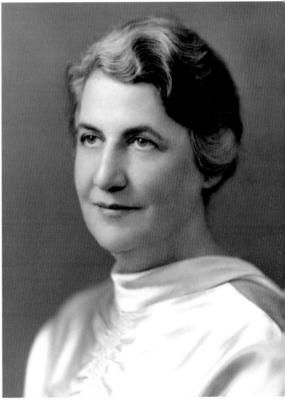

Left: Class of 1927.
Bottom: Director Catherine M. Buckley, 1927–1940.

So great has been the success that the [national] Board of Managers today decided to introduce the system at the central home in Dayton. This home has about 5,500 inmates, almost three times as many as are in the Milwaukee home. The girls for the Dayton home will be secured from

it can be done. I think eventually it will be done in all the homes.—"Doing Good Work: The Female Nurses at the Soldiers' Home Are Commendable by the National Board of Managers," November 12, 1980, *Milwaukee Sentinel*

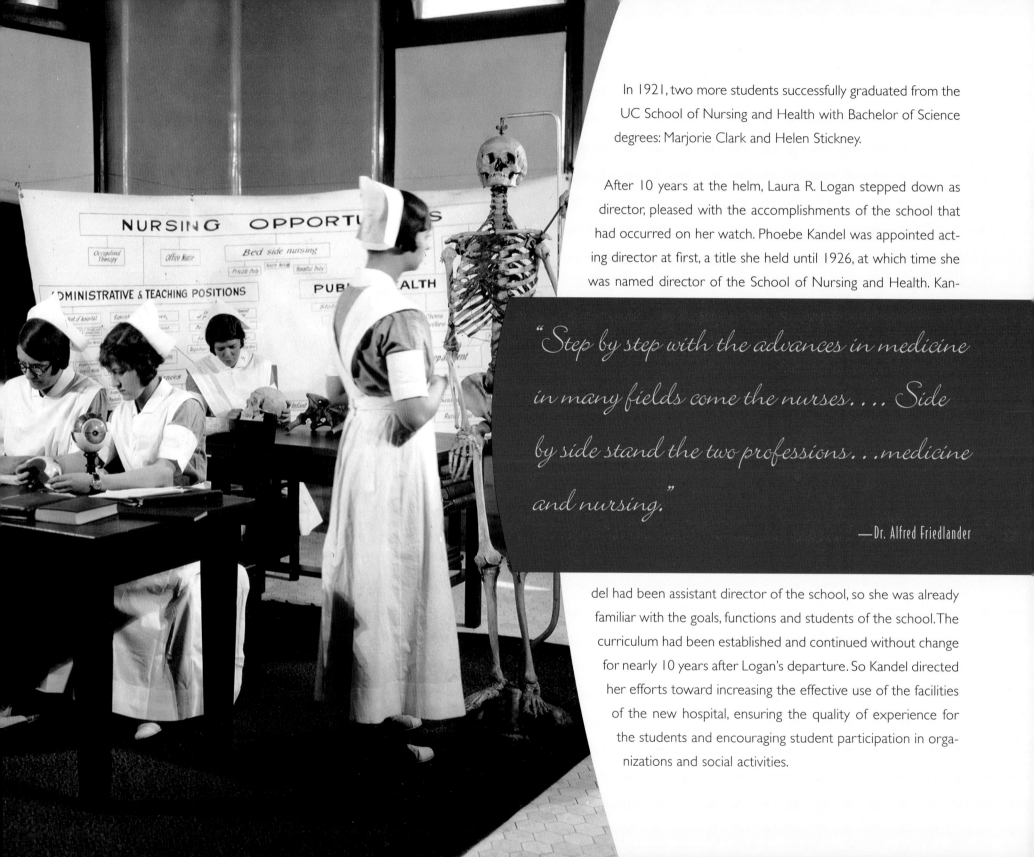

In 1921, two more students successfully graduated from the UC School of Nursing and Health with Bachelor of Science degrees: Marjorie Clark and Helen Stickney.

After 10 years at the helm, Laura R. Logan stepped down as director, pleased with the accomplishments of the school that had occurred on her watch. Phoebe Kandel was appointed acting director at first, a title she held until 1926, at which time she was named director of the School of Nursing and Health. Kan-

> *"Step by step with the advances in medicine in many fields come the nurses.... Side by side stand the two professions...medicine and nursing."*
>
> —Dr. Alfred Friedlander

del had been assistant director of the school, so she was already familiar with the goals, functions and students of the school. The curriculum had been established and continued without change for nearly 10 years after Logan's departure. So Kandel directed her efforts toward increasing the effective use of the facilities of the new hospital, ensuring the quality of experience for the students and encouraging student participation in organizations and social activities.

Although the curriculum was very full and students still had a 48-hour week of clinical hours plus class activities, there was still room for recreation. Some of those included the May Day celebration, Melody Club, Orchestra Association and frequent parties and dances in the Roof Garden of the nurses' home. Students also participated in the school's cooperative student government.

Five students—Hazelle E. Baird, Grace Lloyd, Gladys Shaw Sand, Louise Theobald and Laura Rosnagle (who later became dean of the College of Nursing and Health)—went to the home of Annie Laws to discuss the possibility of starting an honorary professional nursing fraternity, Alpha Alpha Pi. Baird wrote in the *American Journal of Nursing*, "One of the objectives of the Alpha Alpha Pi Fraternity is the furthering of student activities within the School of Nursing and the encouragement of participation in all [university] undertakings." The fraternity was organized in 1924 and became a successful method of encouraging and rewarding high nursing standards, as well as serving as a social outlet for students. This was the first such nursing organization offered on a national basis.

Kandel resigned in 1927, but continued to keep in touch with the school. In fact, in 1950, she donated her own professional collection to the Solomon W. Levi Library to add to the historical collection of nursing materials and books. Her gift was recognized by naming the historical section of the nursing library the "Phoebe M. Kandel Historical Nursing Section of the Solomon W. Levi Memorial Library."

Phoebe Kandel was succeeded by Catherine Buckley. Based on the recommendations of the Goldmark Report of 1923 and the National League of Nursing Education's Standard Curriculum of 1917,

Buckley began her tenure by reorganizing the school and standardizing nursing policy in the hospital and the school. The students still worked many hours in the hospital each week. Hospital nursing service and educational needs were considered equal. However, the number of nurse helpers in the hospital was increased so that the nursing load on student nurses would not be so heavy.

Dr. Alfred Friedlander, dean of the UC College of Medicine from 1935 to 1939, was very supportive of nursing. Speaking to the alumni, he said, "Step by step with the advances in medicine in many fields come the nurses…. Side by side stand the two professions…medicine and nursing." Because of Buckley's hard work, with Dr. Friedlander's support and others, the school was granted full autonomy in 1938.

1920–1929

1924 • The curriculum now included 48 hours of clinical time in addition to classwork.

The first national honorary fraternity, Alpha Alpha Pi, was organized.

Left: Anatomy class in 1928.
Bottom (left to right): Class of 1928, Class of 1929.

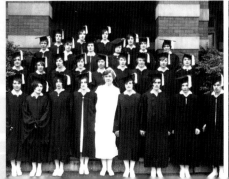

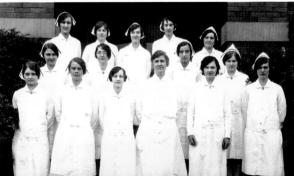

REDEFINING NURSING 1930–1939
Chapter Five

5

At this point in Cincinnati, the Miami & Erie Canal had been drained in 1919 into the Ohio River, so many of the health issues from having an unclean water source running through the middle of town were mitigated. Initially, the bed of the canal was to be used for a subway in Cincinnati. However, with the growing popularity of the automobile, interest in a rail system had waned. The plan was scotched in 1927 in favor of filling in the canal, and in 1928 Central Parkway was dedicated. By this time, though, the hospital had already moved Uptown to Avondale.

Steamboats provided both entertainment and transportation. They also faced their share of trouble. The first Island Queen, a very popular excursion boat ridden by visitors to Old Coney, caught fire in a conflagration at Cincinnati's public landing and burned to the waterline in 1922. (The Morning Star, Island Maid, Chris Greene and Tacoma were completely destroyed in the same fire.)

The Great Depression held the country in its grips, but Cincinnatians were hanging on by a thread. Being fairly conservative, many of the locals had not been putting their money in the banks in the first place. However, the next disaster hit hard: flood.

The great flood of 1937 changed Cincinnati in many ways forever. Because of the city's being on a natural plateau, the flood waters never advanced north of 4th Street. However some businesses, having survived the Great Depression, could not overcome a second blow and were forced to close.

Up until the late 1930s in Cincinnati, most milk was delivered directly to the homes. As the milk men went around to their customers, each customer would indicate how many bottles she wanted that day. In those days, often if the mistress of the house was not home, the milk man would put the milk in her icebox for her. If the milk man didn't sell all his milk that day, he brought some back with him. "Returned milk" was that milk left over in the truck after the day's deliveries. If the milk man still used a horse to get around, that milk stood a good chance of being bad by the time it made it back to the dairy.

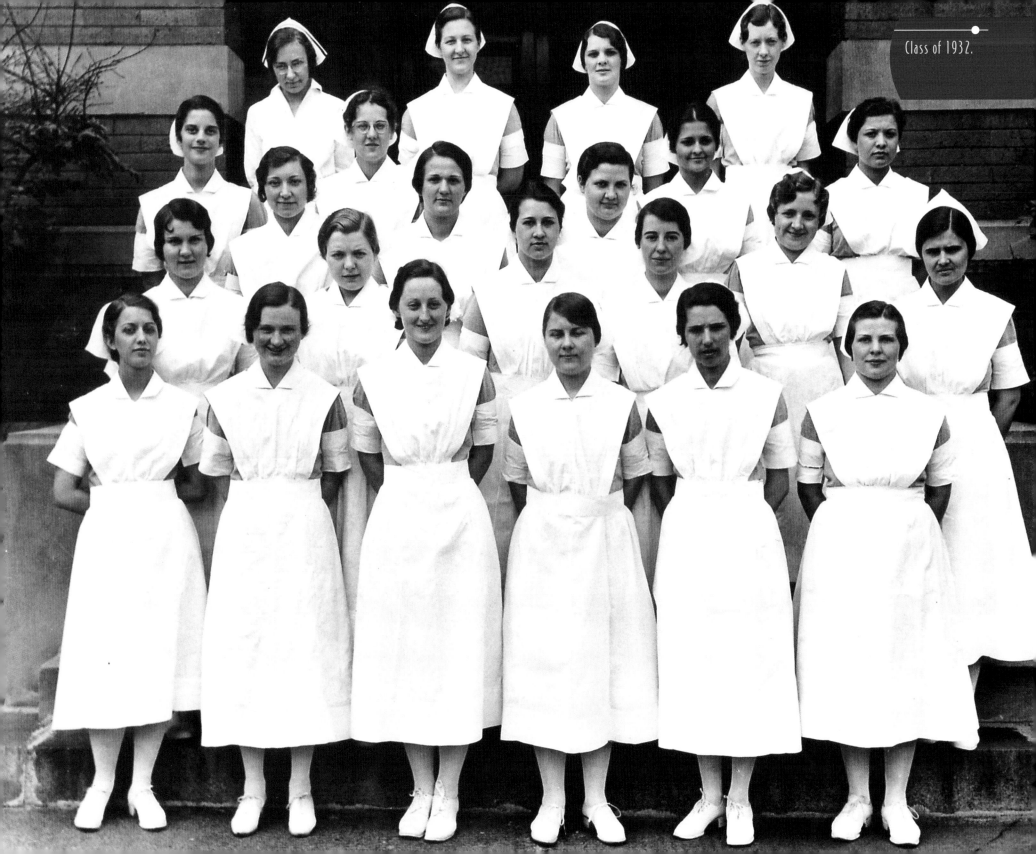

Class of 1932.

During 1932–36, most local dairies phased out their horse-drawn milk wagons and turned to motorized vehicles to make the home

cerned about implementing the new curriculum since a much larger number of students were enrolled in the three-year diploma program

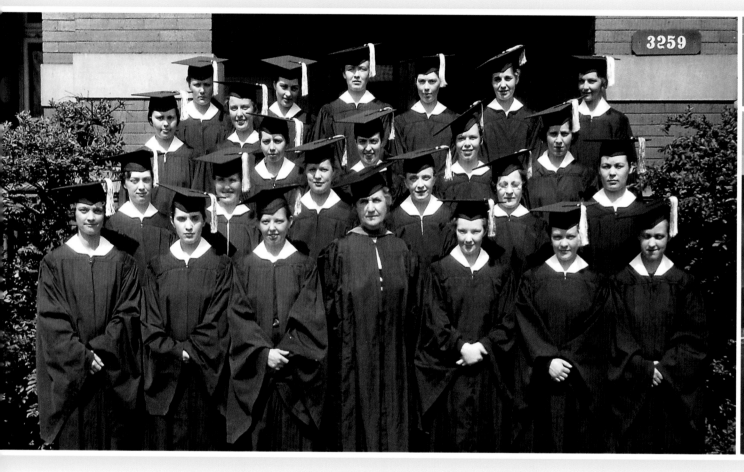

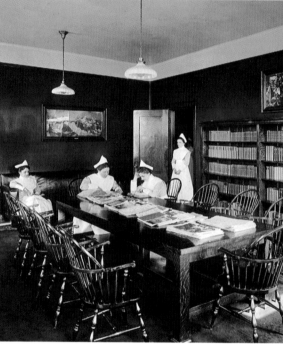

Left: Class of 1934.
Bottom: Logan Hall.

deliveries. It was still unusual for a delivery truck to sell all of its milk. Therefore, the milk that came back had to be tested to see if it was still suitable for use. One of the uses for returns was to separate out the fat and make butter with it.

Also during that time, a four-year curriculum was proposed to replace both the three-year and five-year programs. Many people were con-

than the five-year degree program. Nevertheless, the program offered in 1939 was the four-year program. It was described as follows:

● A combined academic and professional program has been inaugurated, covering a period of four years of three terms each. The length of each term is four months. A month consists of four weeks or 28 days.

● This program begins with an orientation week [that] precedes formal instruction. During this time students are required to take psychological tests, an arithmetic test, physical examinations and a short course relative to study habits. Other functions are arranged, such as excursions through the hospital and the [university] buildings, a student tea, etc.

● Courses taken in the College of Liberal Arts and School of Household Administration during the program include Foods and Nutrition, Introductory Psychology, History, English, Abnormal Psychology, Introduction to the Study of Civilization, Child Development, Public Speaking and Principles of Economics. Students are enrolled for these courses concurrently with the nursing courses…. The non-professional courses in the College of Liberal Arts and the School of Household Administration extend over a period of two terms in each year.

● The first two terms, or pre-clinical period, are devoted largely to the study of the basic biological and social sciences and the Introduction to Nursing Arts. The time is spent chiefly in the classrooms and laboratories of the hospital, College of Medicine, the Pathological Institute, the College of Liberal Arts and School of Household Administration. Experience in the hospital wards is arranged when the student has received sufficient instruction to begin nursing in the hospital.

● During this pre-clinical period the following courses must be satisfactorily completed: Anatomy and Histology, Chemistry, Nutrition, Microbiology, Introduction of Nursing Arts and such other courses [as] may be included.

● During the remaining months of the program, the student begins her regular experience in the various clinical fields and continues her studies in the College of Liberal Arts and School of Household Administration as mentioned above. Instruction is given in the theory of nursing in relation to the various branches of medicine and surgery; pediatrics, obstetrics and gynecology; diseases of the eye, ear, nose and throat; urology; psychiatry; public health and communicable diseases, including tuberculosis. Lectures, classes and ward assignments are so arranged as to make possible satisfactory correlation of theory and practice, and application is made through experience in the corresponding clinical services.

In connection with the medical and surgical services, the pediatric service and the obstetric service, a period is spent in the related clinic in the Out-Patient Department of the Cincinnati General Hospital, where the student has experience in the observation and treatment of ambulatory patients.

This affiliation with the Visiting Nurse Association of the city provides field experience in public health nursing, including observation of programs of school nursing and nursing of families in the home. Physical education is required.

1938 ● The School of Nursing and Health gained full autonomy. The program was changed to a four-year baccalaureate program of general and professional nursing education, and became the eighth college of the university.

1939 ● The four-year program started. Students completing the program received a bachelor of science in nursing degree. The three- and five-year programs were phased out.

GOING TO WAR 1940–1949
Chapter Six

6

The now-autonomous School of Nursing and Health maintained a standard of excellence from its inception. This was accomplished by self-evaluation and curriculum revision. As there was no formal accreditation process for baccalaureate nursing schools prior to 1939, administrators of the school had several agencies evaluate the program. These sources were the National League of Nursing Education, the Association of Collegiate Schools of Nursing, the New York State Board of Regents, the Ohio State Nurses' Board and the United States Cadet Nurse Corps. All granted approval of the UC School of Nursing and Health.

In 1940, when the National League of Nursing Education began an accrediting service, the school applied for the service and was accredited. It is listed on the first published list of national accredited schools of nursing "to give public recognition to schools that voluntarily seek and are deemed worthy of accreditation."

After a long and fruitful tenure, Catherine Buckley resigned in 1940 because of ill health. Helen G. Schwartz became head of the school. In 1943, the school became a college within the University of Cincinnati. The name of the school was changed to the College of Nursing and Health, and the title of dean was conferred upon Helen Schwartz. Faculty members were then listed according to university rank.

Dean Schwartz was prepared to assume the duties of her new position. She had worked as assistant director of the school since 1936. She held bachelor's and master's degrees from Columbia University. She was also aware of national trends because she had worked with the curriculum committee of the National League of Nursing Education and as director of Field Service for the Committee on Nursing Education of the Nursing Council of National Defense.

At the same time that all this was going on within the new college, outside the world was at war. The National League of Nursing Education had recommended that nursing schools consider how students could complete the nursing program in a shorter time to respond to the wartime need for more nurses.

In the summer of 1941, Thomas Parran Jr., the U.S. Surgeon General, asked the University of Cincinnati to organize the 25th General

Hospital Unit to be activated in case of a national emergency. Cincinnati General Hospital had acted in this capacity in World War I. The College of Nursing, in cooperation with the College of Medicine, organized the nursing staff for the unit. It was activated on September 5, 1942. Lieutenant Hattie E. Pugh, assistant professor of the College of Nursing and Health was the Chief Nurse. She was supervisor of Nursing of the Out-Patient Department at Cincinnati General Hospital before leaving with the unit.

Dean Schwartz worked two months on a national project to accelerate basic nursing curricula so larger numbers of nurses could be graduated.

Many other nurses from the college and Cincinnati General Hospital left to serve in the armed forces, thus creating a hardship on those trying to provide direction for students and nursing care for patients. There were 56 officers, 105 nurses (mostly from the Cincinnati area), three hospital dietitians, two physical therapists and 500 enlisted men in the unit. This unit served overseas in Scotland, England, France and Belgium.

Dean Helen Schwartz, 1940-1944.

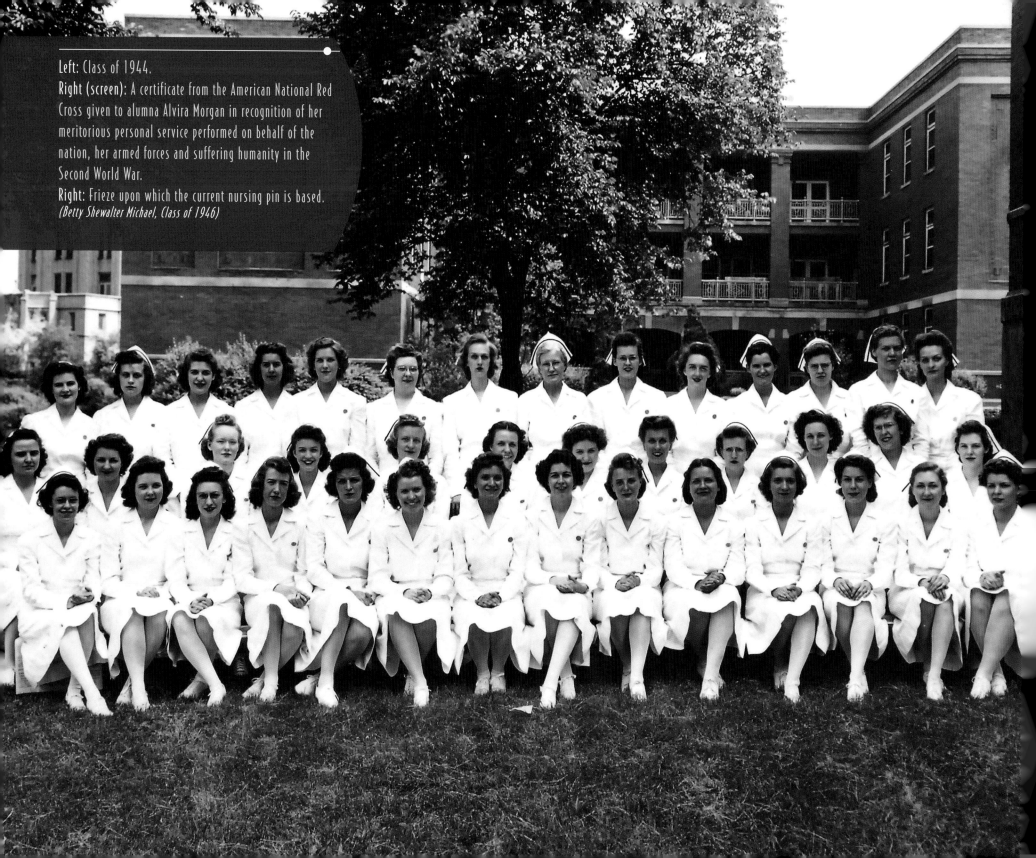

Left: Class of 1944.

Right (screen): A certificate from the American National Red Cross given to alumna Alvira Morgan in recognition of her meritorious personal service performed on behalf of the nation, her armed forces and suffering humanity in the Second World War.

Right: Frieze upon which the current nursing pin is based.

(Betty Shewalter Michael, Class of 1946)

Many nurses in the unit were graduates of the College of Nursing and Health. Bobbie Sterne, mayor of Cincinnati in 1976 and 1979, was not a graduate of UC's College of Nursing and Health, but she did serve as a nurse in the unit.

In the fall of 1942, changes were made in the admission procedures and curriculum to graduate more nurses in less time. These changes included (1) admitting a second class of nurses beginning in January 1943, (2) responding to the Bolton Act of 1943 by becoming a part of the U.S. Cadet Nurse Corps in January 1944, and (3) arranging for the students to complete the nursing courses in a shorter period of time.

Mrs. Frances Payne Bolton was an Ohio congresswoman who had stepped in after her husband had died in office. In so doing, she became the first in the state of Ohio and only the seventh in the House of Representatives. One of her chief political causes was promotion of nursing, nursing education and care of the sick. The Bolton Act created the U.S. Cadet Nurse Corps and appropriated $160 million in federal funds for nursing schools across the country, especially those that educated African Americans.

Dean Schwartz sent a message to the alumni that stated in part, "Effective in [August 1944], a 36-month program of the [college] will be open to two groups. For high school graduates, a Diploma in Nursing will be granted on completion of requirements; for students who presented one or two more years of acceptable college work on admission, a Diploma in Nursing and a Degree of Bachelor of Science in Nursing will be granted. The four year (48 months) combined academic and professional nursing program will be temporarily suspended 'for the duration' for new students." Four-year students already progressing through the program were allowed to complete that program.

This must have been a confusing time for faculty and students. The school was providing a number of different curricula simultaneously.

Faculty also served in many capacities. Dean Schwartz worked two months on a national project to accelerate basic nursing curricula so larger numbers of nurses could be graduated.

After a busy and productive four years, Dean Schwartz resigned in June 1944. Clara Gestel, a teacher in the school since June 6, 1929, was asked to take "Administrative Charge" of the college from April to November 1944. (After the appointment of a new dean, Gestel returned to her previous faculty position and remained with the college until June 1, 1957.)

Laura E. Rosnagle ('26) was officially appointed dean of the College of Nursing and Health on July 1, 1945. However, she had assumed her duties much earlier. She was already very familiar with the school. After receiving her degree from the School of Nursing and Health in 1926, she went on to earn a master's

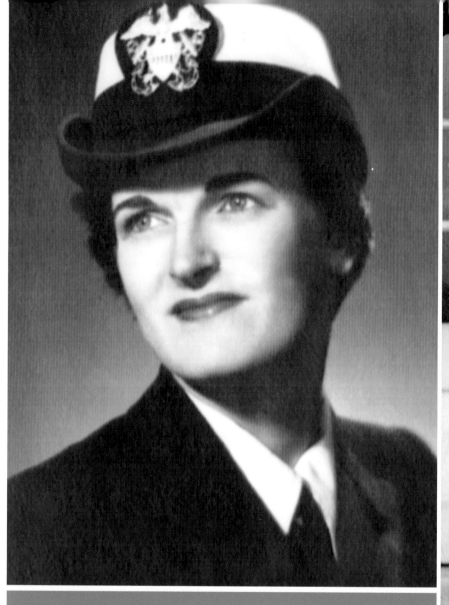

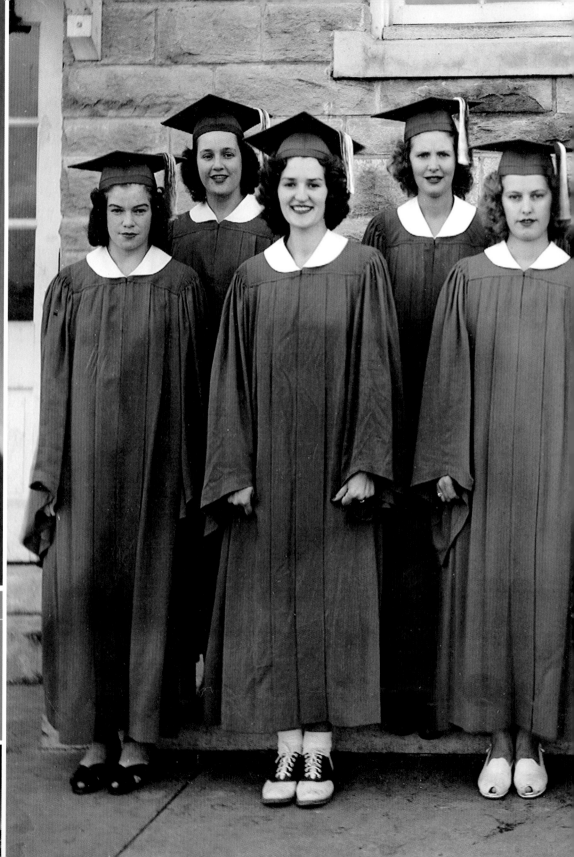

Top: Betty Shewalter Michael (Class of 1946).
Bottom (left to right): Interim Dean Clara Gestel, 1944; Class of 1948.
Right: U.S. Cadet Nurse Corps.

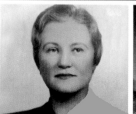

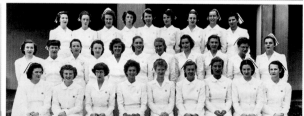

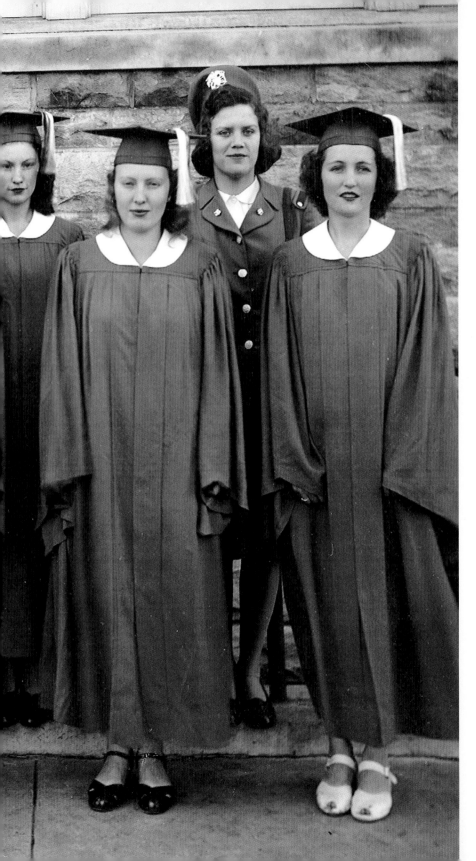

degree from Columbia University. (She was later awarded an honorary LLD from Miami University in 1962.) Dean Rosnagle's prior academic and administrative qualifications included teaching on the faculty of the College of Nursing and Health; the Highland Hospital School of Nursing in Rochester, New York; and the Hartford Hospital in Connecticut.

The lack of supplies and equipment created hardships, but the head nurses, supervisors and students worked to maintain the standards of the College of Nursing and Health.

Many major changes occurred under Dean Rosnagle's leadership. In her doctoral dissertation, Dr. Ruth Moore Bunyan (one of the first three African-American graduates) stated, "Great strides had, in fact, been made at the College in the years [that] spanned the economic depression and the Second World War. Yet, it was evident that in many respects, Miss Rosnagle, as the designated Head of the College, found herself in difficulties very similar to those [that] caused the resignation of Miss Murray, the first Superintendent of the Training School, as she attempted to have nursing education chart its own course."

Dean Rosnagle assumed her new position when the country was just recovering from World War II. Cincinnati General Hospital had insufficient nursing staff and supplies during the war, and this situation continued

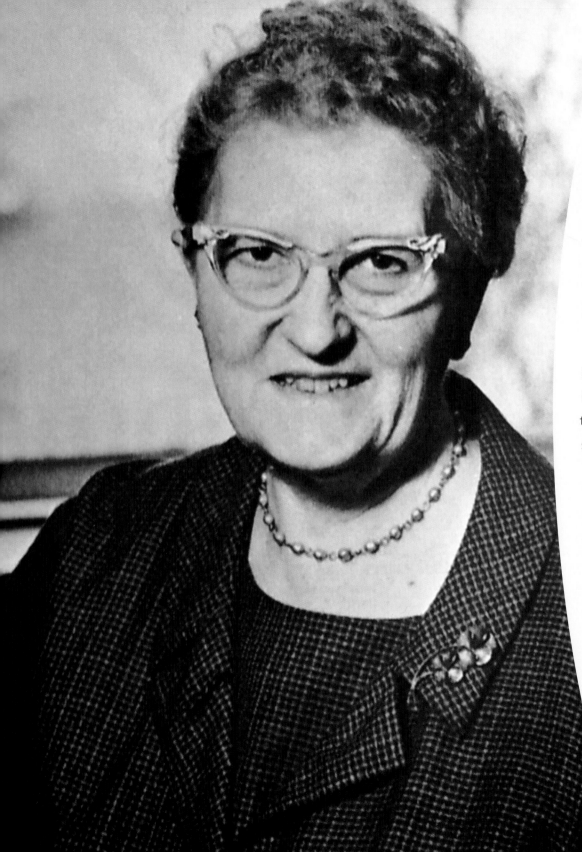

after the war. Nurses spent much more time improvising and borrowing linen and equipment in order to care for patients.

There was a trend to decrease the number of hours that students spent in the clinical area. This was educationally sound but decreased the number of hours that students were available to supply needed nursing care.

Laura Rosnagle noted, "reflecting the social influence, a 48-hour week for students including classes (1937) had gradually been reduced to a 44-hour week in 1948 and a 40-hour week in 1949."

Even with those changes, students still were in the clinical area many hours. The lack of supplies and equipment created hardships, but the head nurses, supervisors and students worked to maintain the standards of the College of Nursing and Health.

There were other changes in clinical times; these were welcomed by the students. Holiday times for students at the College of Nursing and Health were changed so that holidays were observed at the same time as in other colleges. Students would no longer work on Christmas, Easter and other holidays. Many alumni were opposed to these changes, however, believing that students would not have enough time for practicum experience. Other alumni felt that better planning would provide quality experience despite the reduction in clinical hours.

Besides a reduction in clinical hours, there were advances in nursing and medicine. Nurses were beginning to feel a need for more advanced training. One of the dean's goals was to continue to provide instruction and experiences along special lines for people in the community and to develop master's level education for the nurses who were interested. Few such schools existed, and to start such a program was a very complex and expensive process. To accomplish this, efforts were directed toward promoting the concept of graduate education in the community to enlist support and obtain funding.

1940 — The school was accredited by the National League of Nursing (NLN) and became a charter member.

1941 — The United States entered World War II.

1942 — The School of Nursing and Health and the College of Medicine organized the 25th General Hospital Unit. The school became a charter member of the National League for Nursing, the national accrediting agency and has maintained its accreditation without interruption.

1943 — The school became the College of Nursing and Health at the University of Cincinnati with Helen G. Schwartz as its first dean.

1944 — The College of Nursing and Health became a participant in the United States Cadet Nurse Corps.

1947 — The Jane E. Procter endowed Chair of Advanced Nursing Education was established making the UC College of Nursing and Health the first college of nursing to receive an endowed chair.

1948 — The College of Nursing and Health offered programs in pediatrics, psychiatry and advanced nursing theory for registered nurses (RNs).

OFFERING NEW DEGREES 1950–1959
Chapter Seven

In 1950, the College of Nursing was undergoing a great deal of change. Dean Rosnagle wrote, "The present integrated program measurement of suitability is not considered on a time basis but instead, it is determined by the student's ability to continue progressive development. Unquestionably the philosophy of John Dewey of 'experiencing and problem-solving' has had the greatest influence upon education in this period."

Mable I. Darrington described the administrative structure of the college as follows:

> "Laura E. Rosnagle has a dual position as Dean of the College and Director of the Nursing Service in the Cincinnati General Hospital. Assisting her are her two associate directors, Mable I. Darrington, in charge of the Basic Professional Program, and Marcella E. Althoff, in charge of Nursing Service.

> "In the college program, Minnie A. Bohlman is in charge of Instruction in Nursing, Clara E. Gestel in charge of Instruction in Social Sciences and Christine Whitney in charge of Instruction in Biological Sciences. These departments

are organized to include instructors, assistant instructors and junior instructors. The instructors in nursing are Marie K. Freier and Eloise Matthews. Elizabeth Schlegel is an Instructor and Angela Del Vecchio is an Assistant Instructor in Biological Sciences.

"Assisting in the direction of nursing service are Ruby Lapin, in charge of Rotation and Assignments of the students' clinical experiences, and Bertha N. Gordon, in charge of Interdepartmental Relationships....

"Since the clinical experience is equal in importance with classroom instruction in the education of the student nurse, the duties of the supervisors and head nurses are twofold, that of teaching and administration."

A great deal of responsibility rested on the shoulders of a few.

Talking to the Jewish Hospital Board of Trustees about the future of nursing education, Dean Rosnagle noted the need for the availability of advanced professional programs within easy access of every professional nurse. In 1948, through active community interest, money had been provided for an endowed Chair of Advanced Nursing Education to establish programs for graduate nurses. This was the first chair of its kind in the United States. In 1967, the Chair was named for Jane E. Procter.

Authority was given by the Graduate School of the University to the College of Nursing to begin master's programs in pediatrics and psychiatric nursing. A program for diploma registered nurses to work toward a baccalaureate degree was also to be organized. Clara Gilchrist was named Director of Graduate Education and was the first to receive monies from the Chair of Advanced Nursing Education. Both adult and child psychiatric clinical specialist programs were offered at the College of Nursing and Health in 1956. These were among the first such programs to be offered in the country.

The first student to enter the master's program at the college was Patricia Ryan (Wahl) ('55). She graduated June 6, 1958, with a Master of Science in Nursing degree. After graduation, she was hired as an assistant professor to develop the integration of mental health

Korean War Service Medal 50 Years Celebration, 1950–2000, presented to Lois Kern Haber (Class of 1948).

concepts throughout the undergraduate program. She continued to work at the college for many years afterward and became the assistant dean for Graduate Programs.

PROBLEMS IN THE CINCINNATI GENERAL Hospital System

Although the college was an autonomous unit in the university, it remained closely associated with the Cincinnati General Hospital. Students received room and board from the hospital, and clinical instruction was provided by hospital supervisors and head nurses. In return, students gave the greater part of the nursing care in the hospital. Most of the students' clinical experience was at Cincinnati General Hospital, except for time spent at Dunham Hospital of Hamilton County and in public health nursing. Because of the amount of time students were in the Cincinnati General Hospital, the hospital system had a great influence on the quality of clinical experience the school could provide.

Efforts on the part of the city to increase supplies and repair equipment in the hospital were minimal. Information about hospital conditions were given to the city leaders by a few members of the College of Nursing and Health Alumni Association. There were inspections of the clinical area, and after many meetings and much deliberations, funds in excess of $626,000 were released to the Cincinnati General Hospital to improve conditions.

Some of the needed improvements were very basic. For example, up to this time, large blocks of ice were obtained from a tin-lined and paper items; and creating a 20-bed surgical recovery room. The student dormitories were also renovated with a $60,000 allocation.

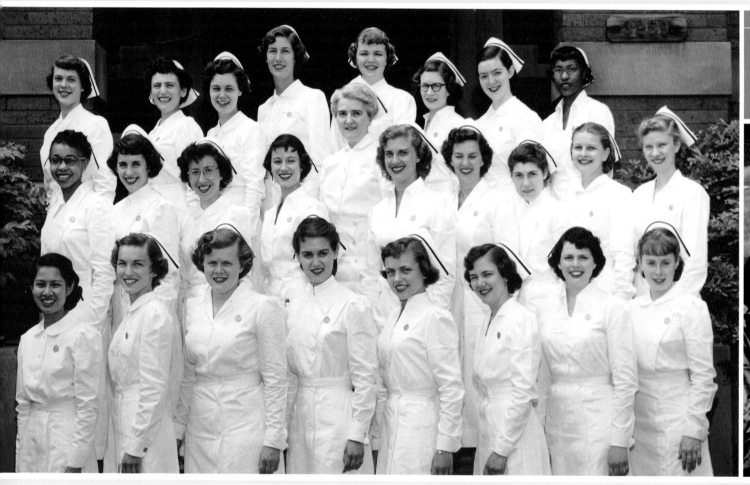

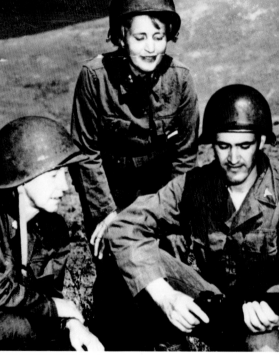

Left: Class of 1951.
Bottom: Major Elsie Grates (Class of 1933).
Photo taken in 1957.

chest standing in the halls outside the wards. When ice was needed, it was chipped off with an ice pick. When funds were given for hospital improvements, this method of obtaining ice was replaced by an electric ice-making machine. Other improvements included enlarging and modernizing Central Sterile Supply; replacing patient furniture; increasing the number of bed linens, medicine glasses, syringes, needles

Other problems with the hospital system money couldn't fix, such as the procedures for determining students' clinical assignments. It was the practice for those assignments to be made by the head nurse, whose primary responsibility was the organization and management of patient care services. When service needs were given precedence, student assignments were not always planned in keeping with the educational

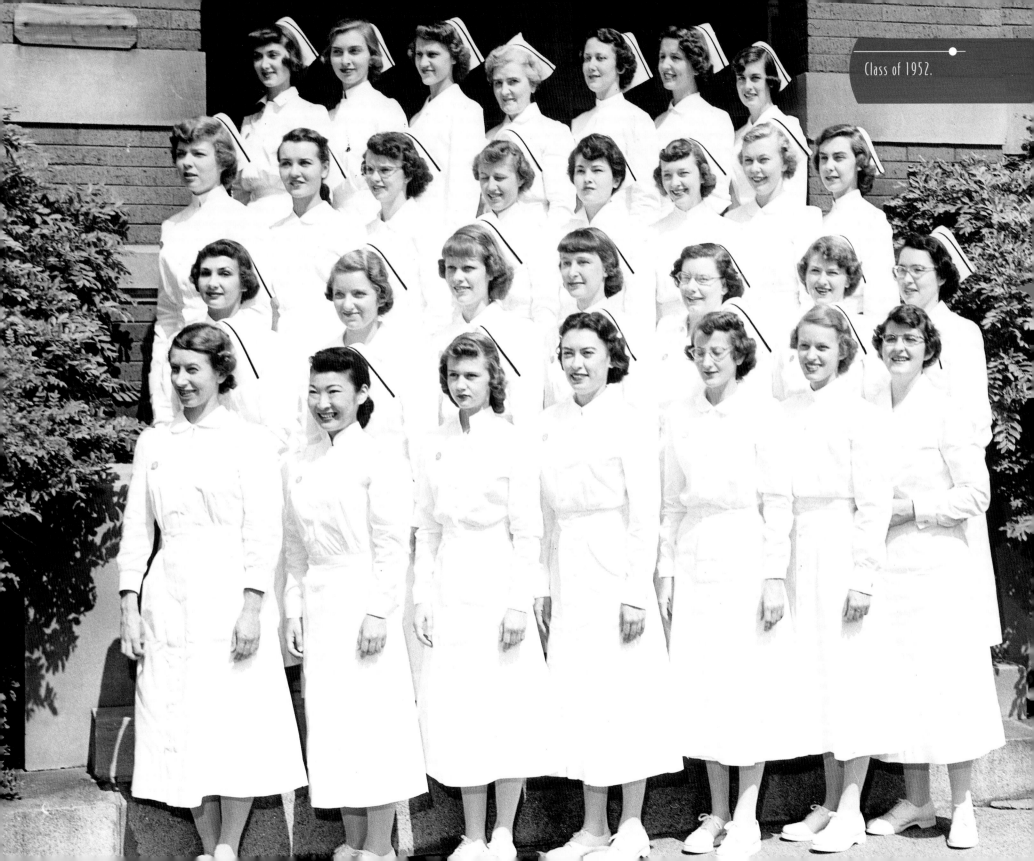

program objectives. Students were frequently assigned to work all three shifts within a week to meet service needs, and they often worked a split shift from 7 a.m. to noon and then 3:30 to 7 p.m. that same day. While this approach was an effective means of increasing nursing service hours, it was clearly detrimental to student learning as it limited time for study.

Data revealed that clinical assignments were frequently made on the basis of service needs, rather than educationally sound principles.

In an effort to resolve these problems, faculty surveyed assignments during the 1953–54 school year. Data revealed that clinical assignments were frequently made on the basis of service needs, rather than educationally sound principles. A constructive outcome of the study was the appointment of an assistant professor who was in charge of the Rotations and Assignments of Students.

During this era, supervisors and head nurses in the hospital were paid by the city and were expected to instruct and evaluate students in addition to carrying out clinical nursing responsibilities. In 1955–56, a Department of Clinical Instruction was approved, and three clinical instructors were hired: Anna Belle Goff, Medical Instructor; Ruth Lingo ('53), Obstetrics Instructor; and Marie Stucker Spruck ('53), Surgical Instructor. These were the first clinical instructors paid by the university. This was the beginning of a fully university-supported faculty at the college.

CHANGES IN THE COLLEGE OF NURSING AND HEALTH— COLLEGE OF MEDICINE— Cincinnati General Hospital Relationships

The Cincinnati General Hospital offered a wealth of experience for student nurses. Many other schools found this to be true and sent affiliating students to benefit from this resource. Still there were many problems. Students continued to work in a service capacity in the hospital; only three clinical instructors were paid by the university; and the dean's responsibilities to the hospital were not clearly defined.

Dean Rosnagle noted in a progress report to the NLN:

"…It may be seen that the complexity of the problem confronting the College of Nursing and Health was not only one of *change of its own program* but one of *change in hospital organization* rooted deeply in the traditions of the past.

"Ours was a complex hospital organization pattern long outdated under which many smarted and fumed but few recognized why or understood its binding control. It hindered progress in many ways.

"To extricate students from the service responsibility for patients in the hospital was to disturb the equilibrium of the entire system on which management and budget of the hospital had been built for *sixty* years."

The dean of the College of Nursing and Health requested to the Board of Directors through the president of the University that the responsibilities of the nursing college to the Cincinnati General Hospital be more clearly defined. Although previously there had been steps toward clarifying the position of nursing in this situation the Board of Directors in February 1956 provided a legal interpretation of the responsibilities of the university for nursing in the Cincinnati General Hospital.

The College of Nursing and Health—Cincinnati General Hospital—College of Medicine relationships were reorganized according to guidelines given by the Board of Directors. It was an involved process generating a great deal of tension. However, changes were made. The responsibilities of the College of Nursing and Health for nursing care at the hospital were placed in line with the responsibilities of the College of Medicine and medical care. Nursing students were no longer placed in a service capacity; clinical faculty were considered university faculty; and the dean of the College of Nursing and Health was clearly responsible to the president of the University of Cincinnati—not the dean of the College of Medicine.

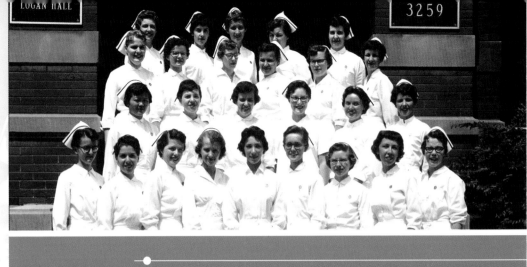

Class of 1957.

1951 — The first and second African-American students were graduated: Arnetta Henderson and Eddie Lee Ralls. The college received charter member accreditation by the National League for Nursing for basic public health nursing content: the 14th college to be so recognized.

1953 — The third African-American student was graduated: Ruth Moore Bunyan.

1956 — The college was among the first colleges to offer the Master of Science in Nursing degree and the first master's student enrolled. Three clinical instructors were hired by the University of Cincinnati. Prior to this, instructors were paid by the city. This milestone marked the beginning of a faculty fully supported by the university. Legal interpretation was established of the responsibilities of the university for nursing in the Cincinnati General Hospital.

1958 — The College of Nursing graduated its first student with a master of science in nursing: Patricia Ryan (Wahl).

1959 — The bachelor of science program changed to four academic years plus two 10-week summer sessions.

EXPANDING COMMUNITY 1960–1969
Chapter Eight

In 1960, the curriculum was revised and organized into clinical fields: (1) medical/surgical nursing, (2) public health nursing, (3) maternal child nursing, (4) psychiatric nursing and (5) foundations of nursing. The length of the program was reduced to four academic years and two 10-week summer sessions. Faculty assumed full responsibility for developing and implementing a curriculum of experiences in nursing.

Laura Rosnagle, in a continued commitment to the community, pursued accreditation in Public Health Nursing for the college. In a presentation to the Women's Club, Dean Rosnagle said, "Public health or community health is such a recent annexation to our thinking that it is badly defined in the minds of the public today."

The Community Health Movement started on an expanded basis only after World War I, principally due to the impetus given by the astounding facts brought to light by the physical examination of young men and women inspected for Army induction. Physical examinations (during World War II) of young recruits were again made and most of the same faults found in young men and women examined in World War I were present in those examined for World War II. These were preventable conditions indicating the need for preventive health programs.

The community health focus that began in 1890 when some of the second-year students were sent out to do district nursing continued. Dean Rosnagle presented a summary of the college's commitment to public health to the Women's Club:

- 1890—Second-year pupils were sent into homes of the community for pay to school (school reimbursed).
- 1894—First graduate nurse employed by Cincinnati Hospital to call on patients who had returned home from the hospital to note their progress and needed care (graduate nurses). Eventually graduate nurses were asked to visit some "needy" patients. As her work increased, the second-year students were permitted to accompany the "visiting nurse" and assist with patient care. Many but not all "pupil nurses" received "home nursing" assignments. This arrangement lasted until 1913.

● 1914—Elective courses of 15 hours in Public Health Nursing were offered in the revised curriculum, including excursions to Health Department, Anti-Tuberculosis League, Children's Clinic and Associated Charities.

● 1915—Three more courses: (1) History and Development of Public Health Nursing in the United States and Abroad; (2) Public Health Nursing Methods; and (3) Teaching Health Principles.

● 1916—Elective excursion plan replaced by "field work under supervision in the various branches of public health."

● 1917—A required block of eight weeks' experience with the Babies Milk Fund Association was established. Included was supervised experience in the Out-Patient Dispensary of General Hospital and its associated subsidiary clinics for child and maternal welfare and observation trips into homes of newborn and sick children.

● 1918—Special eight-month course in Public Health Nursing for graduate nurses was offered.

● 1925—Four weeks tuberculosis nursing practice at Hamilton County Tuberculosis Sanitarium for each student.

● 1938—Experience with Babies Milk Fund Association discontinued; Out-Patient experience was continued and eight weeks with the Cincinnati Visiting Nurse Association (VNA) was arranged, consisting of "field experience, including instruction, observation and participation in various phases of nursing in homes with opportunity to observe programs in school nursing."

● 1942—No Out-Patient or Visiting Nurse Association during the existence of the War-time programs until 1949.

William Cooper Procter. *(Library of Congress)*

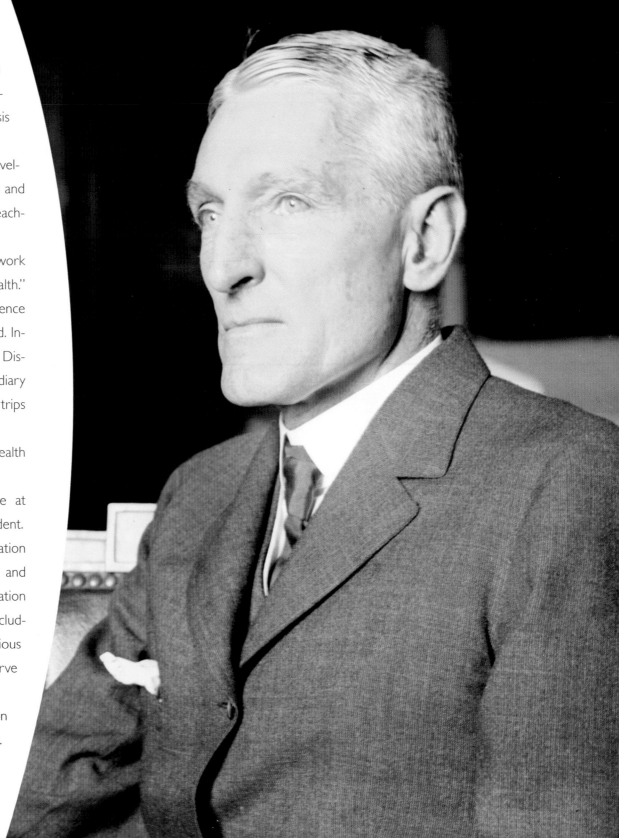

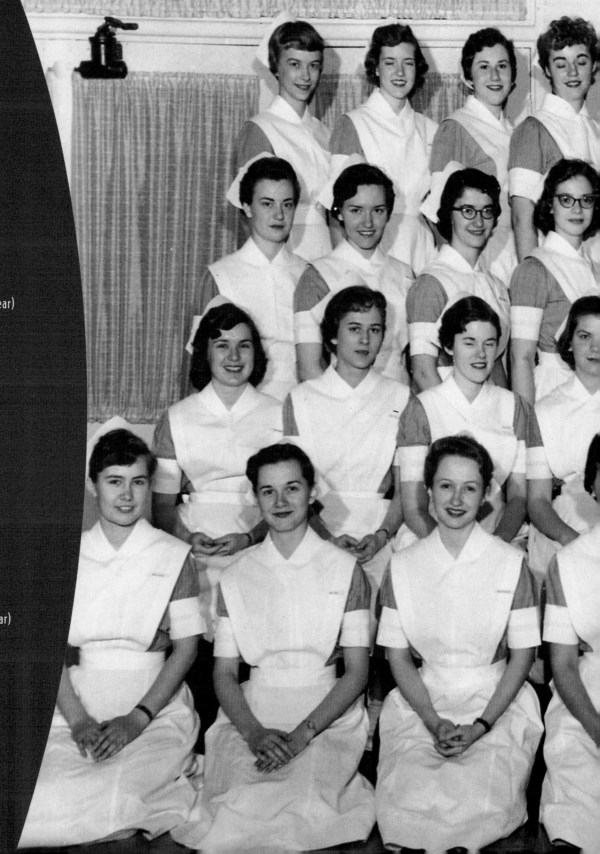

New Curriculum Design

Arrangement of Courses

First Year

English

Western Civilization

Introduction to Sociology

Introduction to Nursing

Basic Science

Physical Education

Summer Session: Clinical Nursing (between second and third year)

Second Year

Nutrition

Introduction to Psychology

Growth and Development

Microbiology

Fundamentals of Nursing

Speech

Third Year

Literature

Introduction to Social Work

History

Clinical Nursing

Summer Session: Clinical Nursing (between third and fourth year)

Fourth Year

Nursing Seminar

Current Problems and Trends in Nursing

Introduction to Public Health

Elective

Clinical Nursing

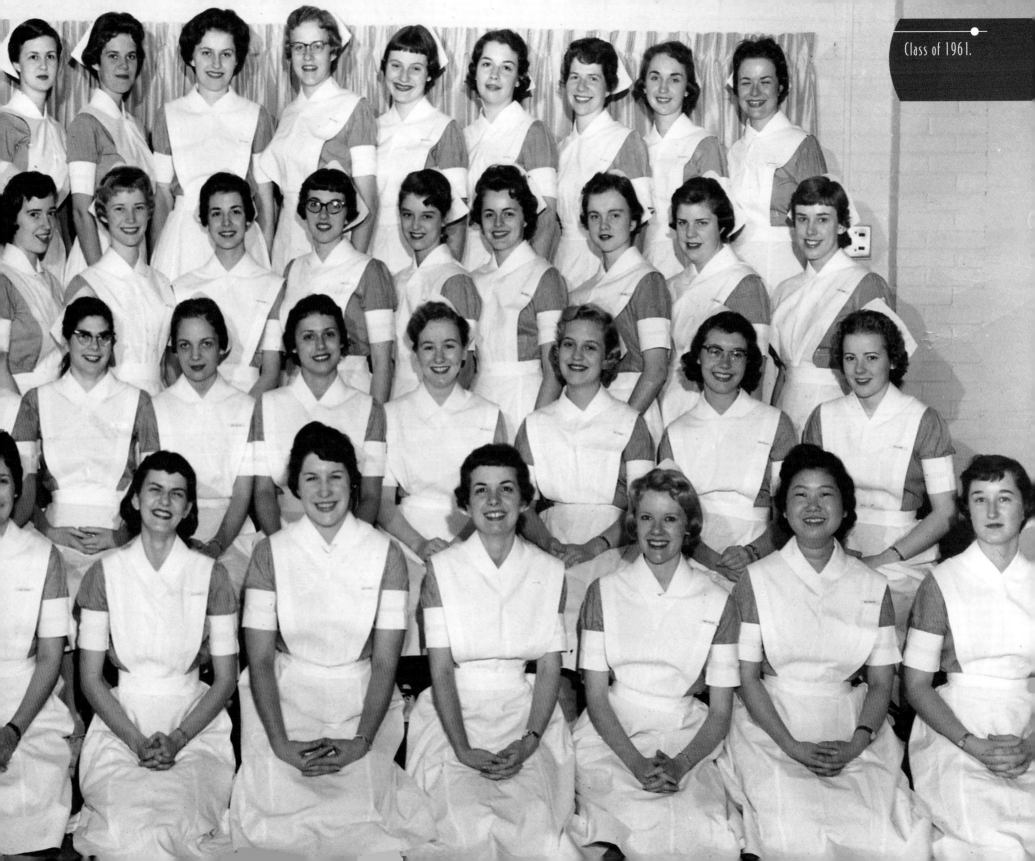

● 1950—Integrated instruction, including practice in applying public health nursing concepts throughout its basic four-year program, planned to include total care of the family as a unit. Field work was transferred from VNA to Cincinnati Health Department. A public health nursing faculty member was employed to give assistance to instructors in the clinical teaching areas and in the agency and coordinate offerings of all areas. Inter-agency referral was initiated.

● 1951—College received accreditation for basic public health nursing—the 14th collegiate school to be so recognized.

● 1958—The first public health nursing field instructor joined the faculty.

● 1960—Concurrent teaching of theory and practice in public health nursing was initiated.

● 1962—The first annual meeting of participants responsible for providing students' learning experiences in public health nursing for College of Nursing and Health students.

As the interest among nurses for advanced education grew, so did the graduate program offerings at the College of Nursing and Health. In keeping with the National League of Nursing accreditation criteria, only those students who held a baccalaureate degree in nursing from an NLN-accredited program were admitted to master's study. The demand for admission to the program was high as the program was the only one available in Southwestern Ohio. As enrollments increased, it became readily apparent that both the human and physical resources of the college needed to be expanded. Plans for a new building were considered.

The Cincinnati General Hospital, built in 1914, with its separate pavilions and connecting underground tunnels was not conducive to the modern system of practicing nursing and medicine. A new hospital was planned. Those planes included using the old hospital for clinics and other services after "renovations."

The new hospital was to be an eight-story high-rise with an emergency unit built between Pavilions B and C. Instructors' offices and conference rooms were to be on each major unit. The old hospital was badly in need of repair and upgrading. In 1960, faculty and students worked in the community to gain voter support for a $17 million bond issue for a new General Hospital and a charter amendment giving full administrative control of the hospital to the university.

In the 1960s, health care was a booming industry requiring an ever-increasing supply of qualified practitioners in all disciplines essential to the delivery of high quality patient care. With the acquisition of Cincinnati General Hospital, it seemed only logical to university administration that the existing health professional colleges and the hospital be organized as a major administrative unit of the institution. Acting upon the following recommendations of a committee that had studied the issue, the University of Cincinnati Medical Center was formed, and Dr. Clement F. St. John was named the first director. Recommendations included the following:

● Transfer full responsibility for management of the Cincinnati General Hospital to the University of Cincinnati;

● The provision at the geographic location of General Hospital of whatever was required in terms of new building equipment and renovation to make the hospital a modern facility for patient care and teaching;

●— Establishment within the university of a suitable organization to manage and correlate the affairs of the Cincinnati General Hospital and the colleges of medicine and nursing in accordance with optimum standards of hospital care and medical education; and

●— The adoption of a sound, long-term plan for financing the operating costs of both the hospital and Medical Center. (The College of Pharmacy became part of the Medical Center in 1969.)

The growth of the College of Nursing and Health after World War II was phenomenal, making it necessary to sequester faculty office space and classroom space in the hospital, the nurses' residence, the College of Pharmacy and numerous buildings on the "Clifton" Campus (what is now called the Uptown Campus). Communication among faculty suffered as it was difficult to locate central meeting places where the faculty could meet to discuss program planning and deal in an organized manner with the day-to-day activities essential to a smooth functioning organization. The need for a facility in which students, faculty and administration could cooperatively work was seen as a high priority of the college.

The alumni, students, faculty and administration approached their many friends for support. In 1963, a donor who wished to remain anonymous contributed a large sum toward the cost of erecting a building to house the College of Nursing and Health. The building was to be called the William Cooper Procter Hall. The new building was to be located at the intersection of Vine St., Martin Luther King Blvd. (the section formerly known as St. Clair Ave.) and Jefferson Ave., midway between the Cincinnati General Hospital and the Uptown Campus.

About the groundbreaking, Dean Rosnagle wrote later, "Dr. Walter C. Langsam, president of the university, outlined the sources of the money which, added to the sizeable grant from the United States Public Health Service (USPHS), made the building possible. Dr. Langsam ably and warmly expressed the gratitude of the university to those who were responsible for bringing the building to reality. Representing the Procter family were Mr. William Cooper Procter's niece, Miss Mary Johnson, two of his grand-nephews, Mssrs. John and Edward Sawyer, and to great-great-nephews, Mssrs. John Pattison Williams Jr. and Alexander Williams. Mr. R. R. Dupree, formerly chairman and now honorary chairman of the Board of the Procter and Gamble Company, and close friend of Mr. Procter during his lifetime, turned the first shovel of dirt for the new building. Representatives from the alumni and faculty of the college, the Board of Directors and university administration, interested community organizations, various schools of nursing and hospitals in Cincinnati and dear friends of the College were in attendance for this happy occasion."

Dean Emeritus Laura Rosnagle retired from the college in 1967 following decades of leadership in the field of nursing. Under her aegis, the college earned its well-deserved reputation for excellence in nursing education. Her wisdom, strength and futuristic outlook are perhaps best captured in her own words: "To say that anything is impossible is ridiculous—yes, even travelling to the moon."

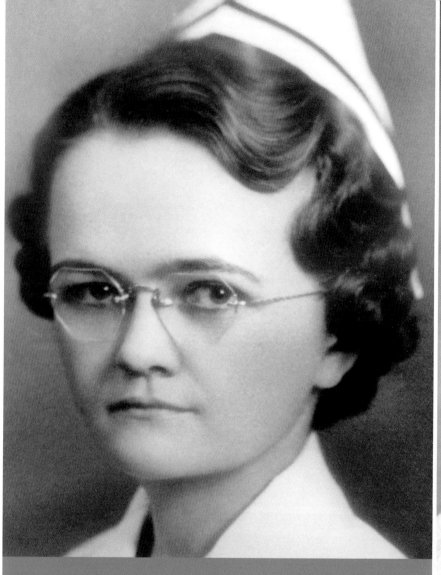

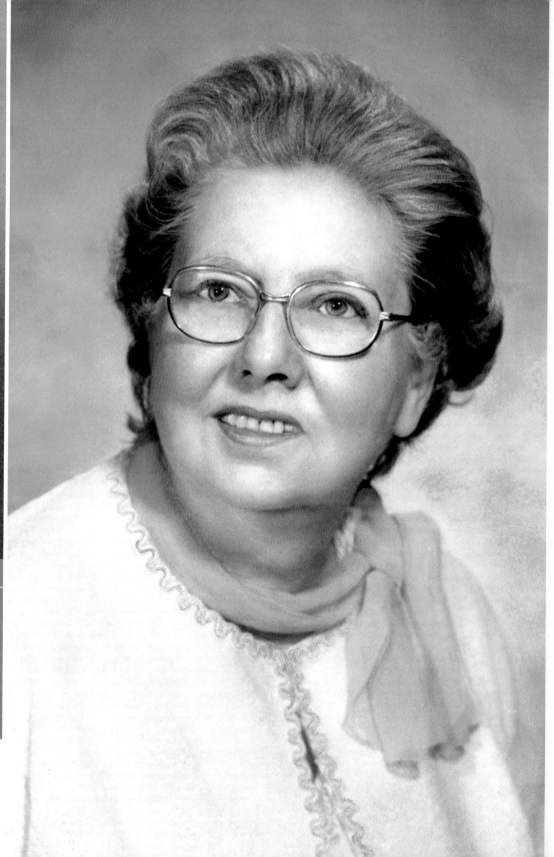

Top: Dean Mable I. Darrington, 1967–1968.
Bottom (left to right): U.S. Navy Captain Susan Stuart Miller (Class of 1966) was stationed in Guam during the Vietnam War and served in Desert Storm; Class of 1968.
Right: Dean Ruth Dalrymple, 1968–1977.

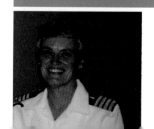

Although retired, Dean Emeritus Rosnagle continued her association with the college for many years, spending time in research, directing the Historical Committee and writing an in-depth history of the school.

A NEW ERA

Assistant Dean Mable I. Darrington became acting dean until a new dean could be chosen. Ruth Dalrymple was appointed dean on August 15, 1967, and assumed the duties of the office on January 24, 1968. Dr. Dalrymple came to the UC College of Nursing and Health with excellent credentials. Her educational background included a Bachelor of Science degree from Muskingum College and a master's degree in nursing, nursing education and administration from Western Reserve University [Case Western Reserve University, as of 1967]. She earned a Doctorate in Public Health at the University of Pittsburgh. She had held positions in nursing service administration and nursing education in Cleveland, Ohio; Richmond, Virginia; and at the University of North Carolina where she was assistant dean of the School of Nursing and director of the Baccalaureate Program. She was also very active in professional organizations. Dr. Dalrymple enthusiastically accepted the position. She had heard of the fine reputation of the College of Nursing and Health and was intrigued by the rich history of the school. One of her first major tasks was to plan the dedication of the new building.

For the first time since the school began in 1889 as the Cincinnati Training School for Nurses, the College of Nursing and Health had the facilities to become a nursing center for the community. The four-story building had space for large administrative and faculty offices, classrooms, conference rooms, the Solomon W. Levi Memorial Library and facilities for a continuing education program. Classrooms had closed circuit television and two-way mirrors. Elevators connected all floors. It was built to accommodate 400 traditional students 100 master's students and 100 students taking continuing education courses.

Dr. Helen Nahm noted the severe shortage of nurses and the significance of the new nursing center to the community of nursing.

In 1967, in the United States, there were only 67,000 nurses with the BSN degree and only 16,000 nurses with a master's degree or higher. There was an ever-present shortage of nurses at all levels. The new building was the realization of a dream of Cincinnati nurses and a response to the societal need for more nurses prepared at the baccalaureate level.

Dean Emeritus Rosnagle was one of the leaders for the building project, spending hours in planning and fundraising. The Better Nursing Committee, an organization of public-spirited Cincinnati women, also provided momentum for planning the building. Many prominent people attended the dedication ceremony on October 10, 1968. Mrs. Phoebe Kandel Rohrer, director of the School of Nursing and

Frances Friedman Schloss has been a member of the UC College of Nursing Board of Advisors since the early 90s. "I was the first member of the board when it was just a germ of an idea," she says. "Dean Andrea Lindell brought the idea of having an advisory board from her former position at Oakland University. It was a wonderful idea because it gave so much more visibility to the University of Cincinnati College of Nursing that it had never had before. It allowed the public to recognize the important role that registered nurses play in the life of medicine—not just the community, but medicine. It gave them status, dignity and an awareness of the unbelievable selflessness of these people."

Schloss has felt passionate about nurses most of her life.

"When I was 10 years old, my beloved grandmother became very ill with Jacksonian seizures and was in a semi-coma for eight years. She was cared for 24/7 by a remarkable team of RNs who were graduates of Good Samaritan Hospital. I was so influenced by their selfless caregiving that they have remained my mentors all my life and I am sure they are the reason I feel compelled to try to help all people in any way I can.",

"I had a great interest also in animals—especially horses and dogs—and we always have them in our family. I was seriously thinking of either becoming a veterinarian or a registered nurse. However, it was war time and I started my freshman year at UC and met and fell in love with my future

husband at the age of 18. He was a senior and went into the Navy upon graduation. I got married at age 19½, just before he left for dangerous overseas duty. So my idea of vet or nursing school never materialized. However I always, as mentioned, had a passion for caring for people. I volunteered for many years working with the Cincinnati Public Schools in the Division of Aid to the Visually Handicapped, handling books on tape, reading service, etc. Tragically, my passion of helping people was put to the test when my first husband was stricken with midlife diabetes and Lou Gehrig's disease [amyotrophic lateral sclerosis (ALS)] in his early 50s. We spent a great deal of time at the National Institutes of Health in Washington. He had 14 admissions in all. And being the remarkable person he was, he knew there was no cure for this intractable disease, so he wanted to let NIH do experimental treatment so others in the future might benefit."

"During his illness, I was privileged to meet one of the professors from the College of Nursing, Ida Horvitz, who became fascinated with the intensive care unit I ran in my home. She encouraged me to write a manual on taking care of the terminally ill, which I did. This manual is still used by many colleges. It was also videotaped and the video is still used today.

Schloss remarried after her first husband died. Some 20 years he developed pancreatic cancer, and her coping and caring were, sadly, put to use again.

Schloss has received many honorary awards for her work with the visually impaired and for caring for the terminally ill. For example, in 2008 she received the Caring Award from the Visiting Nurse Association.

"My raison d'être for my association and advocacy of nursing and nurses relates to the bottom line of health care: that is the patient. So many students graduating today want to go into research and teaching and forget the true heart of nursing—care of the patient at the bed side. True patient nursing must be given more recognition and these nurses who are on the floor and in the ER and intensive care and surgery must be given equal status with professors and researchers. Nursing is a fine, satisfying career with new and exciting improvements all the time and it offers so many varied opportunities that make it so important to keep nursing contributions to every community alive and visible. Everyone wants to be big in research and teaching, but without the patient you don't need research. Bedside nursing must not be forgotten!"

Health from 1925 to 1927 was one of those present for the community celebration.

Dr. Helen Nahm, dean of the University of California San Francisco School of Nursing, gave the dedicatory address. She spoke about those who questioned the relevance of university offerings and the unrest in the world—for the United States was involved in the Vietnam conflict at the time. She also noted the severe shortage of nurses, especially those who were baccalaureate prepared and the significance of the new nursing center to the community of nursing. She was awarded an honorary Doctorate of Humane Letters.

SOCIETAL CHANGE
AND ITS EFFECT ON
America

Dean Dalrymple had assumed a leadership role at the college during one of our country's most dynamic times of domestic unrest and involvement in violence abroad: the Vietnam war, the Kent State incident, students demanding reform in education, African Americans demanding equal rights, rioting in the streets in Cincinnati and other major American cities, and women re-examining their own traditional roles.

The Rev. Dr. Martin Luther King Jr. felt that racial reform in the United States was being destroyed by the Vietnam War because all the monies were being spent on the war. He noted that there was little left for social reform. The assassinations of President John F. Kennedy, Senator Robert F. Kennedy and Dr. King occurred during these turbulent times.

There was also a great deal of administrative change at the university at this time. Three presidents were appointed between 1968 and 1977: Dr. Walter C. Langsam, Dr. Warren Bennis and Dr. Henry Winkler. There were also changes in the administration at the Medical Center as the university moved from a private and city-financed institution to a state-supported institution.

The new dean had the responsibility of dealing with society and academic changes while directing education at the College of Nursing and Health toward something that would be relevant for the 21st century. She was convinced that nursing would be very different at that time and that the school must be prepared to give students an education that prepared them for this new era.

In response to community needs, a full-time Continuing Education Program was established at the college in 1968 to offer non-credit workshops and short-term courses taught by an interdisciplinary faculty. This reinforced the concept of sharing social and professional responsibilities with others. The college was the first school in the state to establish such a program. Ida Horvitz, assistant dean of Continuing Education in 1968, estimated that during the first 20 years of the program's existence, it provided well over 1,000 programs and workshops to 35,000 health professionals.

Before Dean Dalrymple arrived, the faculty and Dean Rosnagle had been working very hard on a major curriculum revision. The work continued with an increased emphasis on community and family. The first class in the new curriculum entered in 1969. The length of this program was changed to four academic years plus one summer session. The curriculum was developed on the concept of four levels Level I included the Freshman and Sophomore years; Level II, the Junior year; Level III, the Senior year and Level IV, graduate education.

Skills laboratories in Procter Hall were developed and used to help students learn nursing procedures before going to the clinical area. These were an essential part of student learning. One of the areas emphasized in the curriculum was the well family. Each student was assigned one family in the community. The students made home visits to their families on a regular visits, beginning the sophomore year. Faculty often supervised these visits.

Other changes made to the curriculum were made in recognition of the needs of minorities at the university and in the community. Some of the changes included adding courses related to race relations and Black History, and placing more books about the African-American population, its history and concerns in the libraries. Increased efforts were directed toward the recruitment of minority personnel and students.

Efforts at the college were also directed toward assisting the educationally disadvantaged ethnic minorities. Modest financial assistance was obtained through the Sealantic Fund provided by John D. Rockefeller Jr. to which Doris B. Clement was appointed as the Sealantic

Fund Coordinator. She came well prepared for this position having a bachelor's degree in nursing and a master's degree in education with a major in guidance and counseling.

The program was established to help junior and senior high school students develop skills that would enable them to qualify for admission to nursing programs. Some students were involved in the program for as long as four years. The program encompassed two major areas of assistance: academic guidance and remedial work. Clement worked though appropriate channels within the public school system to identify educationally disadvantaged students interested in nursing. Many students benefitted from this program. This was the first of its kind at the University of Cincinnati for disadvantaged youth. It was later phased into the Project for Youth and Upward Bound Program.

1960 — The university was given control of Cincinnati General Hospital by the city of Cincinnati.

1961 — The Cincinnati Medical Center formed, composed of three colleges: Nursing, Medicine and Pharmacy.

1963 — The semester system was changed to a quarter system for the entire university.

1964 — Students entering the program now had to pay board. It was no longer furnished by the Cincinnati General Hospital system.

1966 — Groundbreaking for William Cooper Procter Hall was held. William Cooper Procter had been the son of Procter & Gamble founder, William Procter. The College of Nursing was the first nursing school in the United States to have two endowed chairs with the addition of the Jacob G. Schmidlapp Chair of Nursing, to be occupied by the dean of the college.

1968 — William Cooper Procter Hall (at the corner of Vine St. and what is now Martin Luther King Blvd.) was dedicated. The College of Nursing and Health moved to its current location in Procter Hall, the first independent facility on UC's campus dedicated to the education of practitioners of nursing. The Continuing Education Program was established the same year.

CHANGING THE FACES OF NURSING

Chapter Nine

9

To create a school where equal consideration was given to all groups equally, an Affirmative Minority Action Program was developed. This followed the mandate of the Amendment to the Civil Rights Act of 1972, which prohibited discrimination due to race, religion, sex, color or national origin in public land, private institutions or higher education.

In 1975 the college received a grant from the Center for Minority Affairs of the National Institute of Mental Health to start the Minority Nurse Recruitment Training and Manpower Program. The college could recruit and admit 65 talented minority students. This was believed to be the largest grant ever awarded for a minority program in one discipline up to that time. The first-year award was for $155,000 with $139,325 awarded for each of four subsequent years.

The purpose of the program was to devise and implement strategies to increase the skills and number of minorities engaged in psychiatric mental health. Efforts were directed toward facilitating the admission process and initiating courses designed to increase the knowledge of minority value systems and lifestyles. Relationships between minority and majority groups were considered with emphasis on particular mental health problems associated with minority lifestyles. Workshops were provided on a regular basis to increase faculty understanding of and appreciation for minorities.

Twenty students were admitted into the program the first year. Students were taken into the undergraduate or graduate program and given needed support to succeed. Carolyn Carter was appointed Project Director. She devoted many hours to support activities to promote the success of every student in the program.

STUDENT AND FACULTY Unrest

Student unrest was greatly influenced by the Kent State University tragedy on May 4, 1970, in which Ohio National Guardsmen killed four unarmed college students. As with many other campuses across the country and especially in Ohio, this incident had an inflamma-

The closing of the school created many problems. Students were unsure as to whether or not they would be able to graduate and were

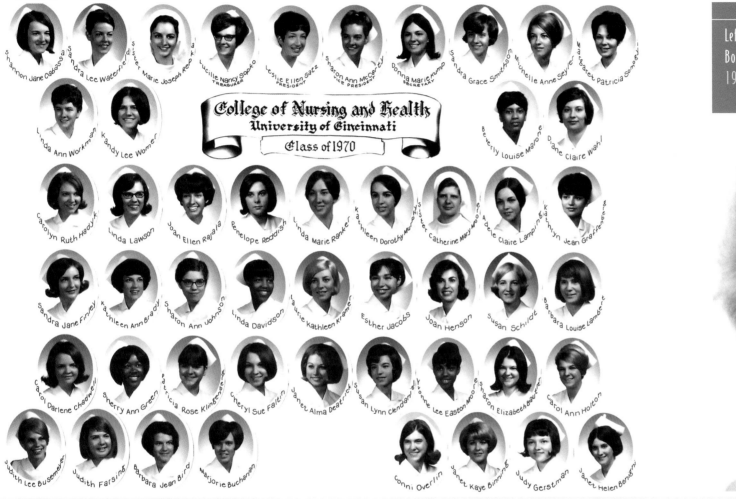

College of Nursing and Health
University of Cincinnati
Class of 1970

Shannon Jane Cabassa
Sandra Lee Waterfield
Sister Marie Joseph Repp
Lucille Nancy Sopko TREASURER
Leslie Ellen Satz PRESIDENT
Sharon Ann McCarty VICE PRESIDENT
Donna Marie Krump SECRETARY
Sandra Grace Smithson
Michelle Anne Seyler
Margaret Patricia Somogyi

Linda Ann Workman
Kandy Lee Womer
Beverly Louise Malone
Diane Claire Wahl

Carolyn Ruth Hadjuk
Linda Lawson
Joan Ellen Rajala
Penelope Reddish
Linda Marie Ranker
Kathleen Dorothy Mullis
Sister Catherine Mary Moeller
Adele Claire Lampin
Kathryn Jean Graffenberg

Sandra Jane Finley
Kathleen Ann Brady
Sharon Ann Johnson
Linda Davidson
Laurie Kathleen Kramer
Esther Jacobs
Joan Henson
Susan Schildt
Barbara Louise Lambert

Carol Darlene Chadwell
Sherry Ann Green
Patricia Rose Klingenberg
Cheryl Sue Faltin
Janet Alma Deatrick
Susan Lynn Clendaniel
Yvonne Lee Easton
Sharon Elizabeth Moore
Carol Ann Holton

Judith Lee Busemeyer
Judith Farsing
Barbara Jean Bird
Marjorie Buchanan
Conni Overlin
Janet Kaye Binning
Judy Gerstman
Janet Helen Benigni

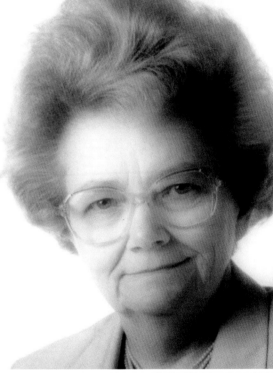

tory effect on the student body at the University of Cincinnati. To prevent the possibility of injury to anyone, the campus was closed two times in the spring quarter of 1970. The second closure was for the remainder of spring quarter.

even more anxious about whether or not they could pass State Boards. (Some students didn't receive their physical degrees until 40 years later, when the university held a special commencement for those who never "graduated.") There was also unrest among the faculty who felt they were being unfairly treated by university administration. The issues were insurance and wages. But the college and the university worked through it.

MERGING OF Honoraries

The honorary fraternity Alpha Alpha Pi had been started at the college in 1924 and had since then continued to support excellence in nursing. Dean Dalrymple, a charter member of Case Western's Sigma Theta Tau, felt that a merger between the two would benefit both students and faculty. The purposes of Sigma Theta Tau were to

- Foster high professional standards;

- Encourage creative work;

- Promote the spirit of fellowship among members of the profession of nursing;

- Promote the maximum development of the individual and thus increase ones capacity to serve the profession and, through it, society;

- Develop an abiding interest in the advancement of nursing; and

- Promote continuous participation as responsible members of the profession.

After much planning and collaboration with officers and members of both honoraries, the college became the Beta Iota Chapter of Sigma Theta Tau in 1972.

FINANCIAL SUPPORT Plummets

In the mid-70s, university fiscal problems forced President Bennis to mandate a nine percent reduction in college budgets. This reduction had serious implications for the college as undergraduate student enrollments were at a new high and the demand by the community for additional graduate programs was increasing. Budget reductions also had a negative impact on the dean's ability to recruit well-qualified faculty. It soon became evident that new program development could not occur unless external funds were obtained.

With Dean Dalrymple's able leadership, the faculty responded to the challenge. In 1974, a master's program to prepare clinical nurse specialists in gerontology was developed from grant monies. This program was in response to a community need since there was an increasing number of elderly people in Ohio. In fact, the number of elderly in Ohio was very close to the elderly population in Florida. This program was the only one of its kind in this area of the country. The following year a federal-funded program to prepare Clinical Nurse Specialists in burn and trauma nursing was also implemented.

Although the students in the school were provided observational experience in industry as early as 1914 and were given courses that included industrial nursing content in 1916, it was not until much later that a program was established to prepare occupational health nurses. In 1976, a master's program to prepare Occupational Health

Nurse Clinical Specialists was developed and offered through the college. This program was funded by the National Institute of Occupational Safety and Health (NIOSH) in an effort to prepare professionals to protect the health of the working individuals or increase the skills of nurses who were already working in occupational health nursing. It was a school in the first Education Resource Center in the United States.

The success of the faculty in obtaining external funds made it possible to expand the graduate program and to redirect general funds to support the growing undergraduate program. During this period, applications to the undergraduate program numbered well over five hundred. In response to demand, the size of the freshman class was increased to 150 students—the largest class ever.

With the increased numbers of undergraduate and graduate students, finding space in clinical facilities was often difficult. Many schools were competing for the same space. The Cincinnati General Hospital could no longer serve as the principal clinical facility for College of Nursing and Health students. Community hospitals, the Veterans Administration Hospital, Cincinnati Children's Hospital, Longview State Hospital and occupational health settings, as well as many other health care agencies were used as practice sites. The expansion of clinical sites provided opportunity for students to work with patients from all socioeconomic levels in a variety of settings. While the concept of variety was educationally sound, it did place an added burden on the faculty who were now required to travel extensively in order to instruct and supervise students in multiple clinical sites.

INTER-AND INTRADISCIPLINARY
Innovations

As the university and its constituent components grew in size and complexity, communication between and within disciplines suffered. The need to develop a closer relationship between nursing education and nursing service at the Medical Center in order to prepare students for practice in the real world of health care delivery became very apparent. To achieve this goal a new position with a triple focus was created by Dean Dalrymple. Mary Ann Mikulic practiced as a clinical specialist with Dr. Jebsen, taught at the college and acted as a Rehabilitation Nurse Consultant throughout the hospitals of the Medical Center.

There was also some experimentation with joint appointments. Faculty members in these positions were expected to spend equal time at the college and at Cincinnati General Hospital. The experiment was not without problems, however, as faculty were not always successfully able to balance the demands of patient services and student instruction while engaging in research and other scholarly pursuits. Eventually expectations for this dual type of role were modified and selected joint appointments for the College of Nursing and Health in the College of Medicine and in nursing service at University Hospital continued.

In 1973, the university introduced a formal process of administrative and faculty review. Dean Dalrymple was an advocate of constructive, evaluative review as a means of maintaining institutional quality. In order to gain acceptance of the process by the faculty and staff, she requested that she be the first person reviewed. In October 1973, the Periodic Review Committee unanimously recommended to Dr. Edward Gall, Vice President and Director of the Medical Center, that Dr. Dalrymple be reappointed as dean. Annual evaluations and periodic review are now standard operating procedures in the college.

In 1977, Dr. Dalrymple relinquished the position of dean. She remained on the faculty in a teaching position to facilitate the transition to a new administration, however. She retired from the college in 1980 as dean emerita.

During the time the new dean was being sought, Dr. Rosalie Cockerill Yeaworth ('51, '66), assistant dean of the graduate program, served as acting dean from September 1, 1977, to August 1, 1978. Following the appointment of the new dean, she returned to her former position. She resigned the following year to become dean of the School of Nursing at the University of Nebraska in Omaha.

Upon Dean Dalrymple's announcement, a nationwide search was begun to find the most qualified person to serve as dean of the College of Nursing and Health. The Search Committee was charged with recommending a leader in nursing education and administration who would advance the goals of the college in the coming decade. From the many applicants and nominees, the committee recommended a woman from New York whom they believed had the credentials to meet the challenge. This well-qualified nominee was Dr. Jeannette Spero.

A graduate of the Bellevue Hospital School of Nursing, Dr. Spero went on to earn her baccalaureate, master's and doctoral degrees from New York University and the Master of Public Health degree from Johns Hopkins school of Hygiene and Public Health. While completing her formal education she also attended the University of Oslo Norway, and the University of Rio Piedras in Puerto Rico for advanced study in public health.

Dr. Spero held the positions of department chairman, acting academic dean and dean of the school of nursing at the State University of New York at Buffalo. Before relocating to Upstate New York, Dr. Spero served as the director of the Graduate Programs in Community Health Nursing at New York University. Earlier in her professional career, she was employed as a hospital staff nurse and as district supervisor of the Visiting Nursing service of New York.

Although offered the position in March 1978, the new dean was unable to relocate until September as her husband, Dr. Herbert S. Rabinowitz, had to find a new position in Cincinnati and her youngest son had to complete his senior year in high school. The Search Committee was impressed with her credentials, her positive outlook and her philosophy of nursing education, and was willing to wait until she was available to take the position. She served as consultant to Acting Dean Yeaworth until official appointment as dean in September 1978.

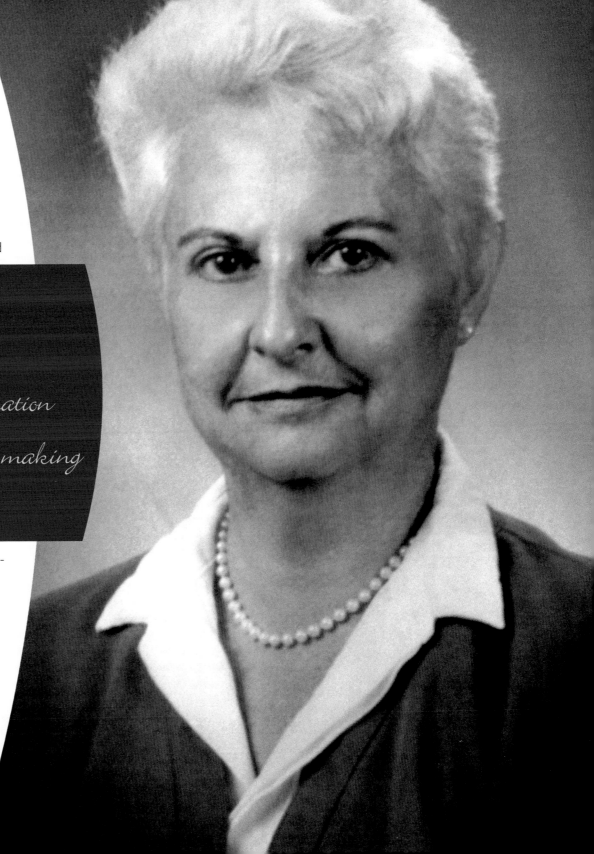

GOALS BASED ON
Assessment

At the first meeting of the Faculty Organization the new dean shared her perceptions of the status of the college and solicited faculty suggestions directed toward reinforcing perceived

It was clear to the new dean that an atmosphere of openness, trust and accountability by fully sharing information and encouraging participatory decision-making had to be created.

strengths and eliminating perceived weaknesses. Identified positive attributes were:

● — a strong history of unique contributions to nursing and nursing education;

● — a small but active cadre of loyal alumni;

● — a stable faculty open to redirection and change;

● — an enthusiastic student body involved in the governance of the college;

Dean Jeannette R. Spero, 1978–1990.

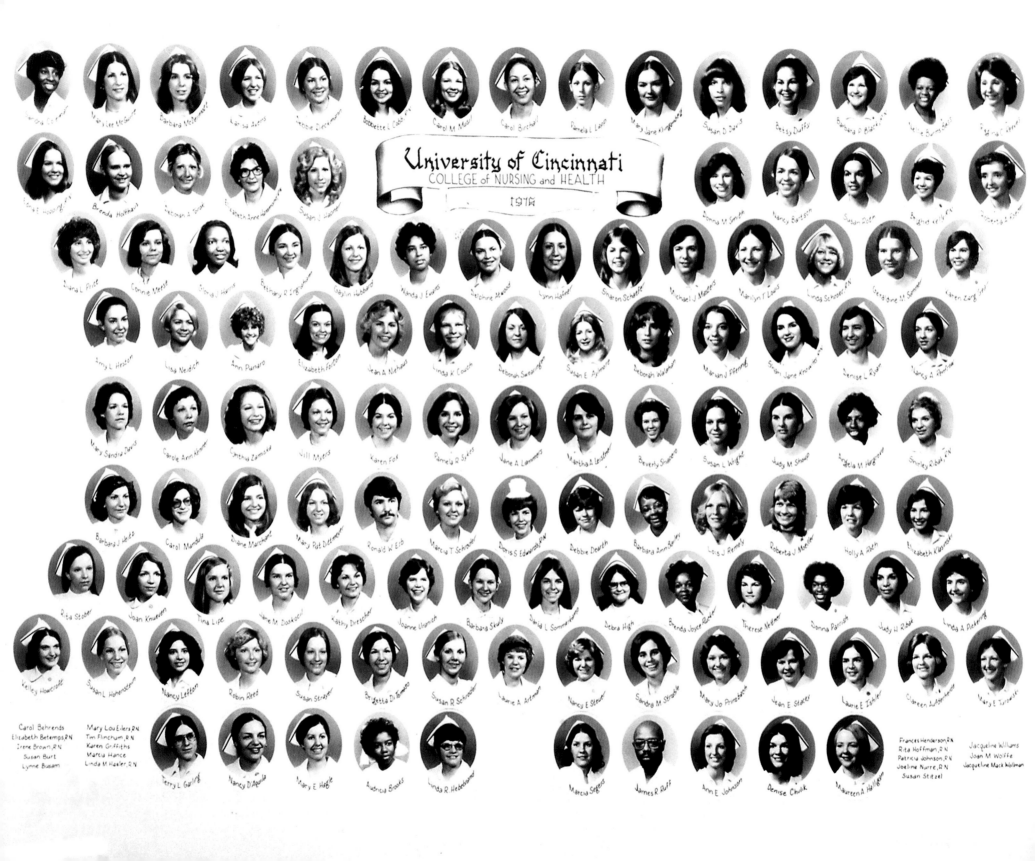

University of Cincinnati
COLLEGE of NURSING and HEALTH
1978

access to excellent clinical facilities;

• stable endowments that provided some budgetary flexibility; and

• recognition by university administration of the vast potential of the college, coupled with a declaration of administrative support.

Less positive attributes to which immediate attention needed to be directed included:

• a weak General Funds support base with approximately 68 percent of the graduate program operating budget derived from soft money that was earmarked for termination;

• anticipated elimination of federal "capitation" dollars that were used to support the student Learning Resource Center;

• a relatively low level of intra- and interdisciplinary interaction fostered by the physical, psychological and political isolation from the mainstream of the university and Medical Center;

• low faculty morale relative to perceptions of unfair treatment by university administration in matters of wages and benefits; and

• a paucity of faculty prepared at the highest educational level expected in academia.

The dean and faculty identified several immediate, intermediate and long-term objectives and began to plan together for their implementation. Short-term objectives were directed toward improvement of faculty morale and adjustments in fiscal resources. Intermediate ob-

jectives addressed faculty development, curriculum revision and enhancement of intra- and interdisciplinary relationships. Long-term objectives were identified as development of a doctoral program, building expansion to house a Center of Nursing Research and the acquisition of a third endowed chair in recognition of the 100th anniversary of the college 10 years hence. (The third endowed chair objective was not attained in time for the 100th anniversary.) All objectives led toward the goal of increasing the college's visibility within the university and the local, state and national community.

Collective bargaining is now an established norm at the University of Cincinnati.

Sensitive to the feeling of the faculty Dean Spero believed that little constructive change could be accomplished in the college until attention was given to the issue of faculty morale. In an effort to discover if consensus existed on particular "morale" issues, the faculty agreed to anonymously respond to an objective questionnaire. Analysis validated the existence of a problem. It was clear to the new dean that an atmosphere of openness, trust and accountability by fully sharing information and encouraging participatory decision-making had to be created if faculty were to develop a sense of pride in themselves as well as in the college. Initiatives included reassessment of responsibilities revision of procedures and policies and creation of new faculty/student committees to provide direction for internal activities as well as activities that interfaced with the external community. The College of Nursing and Health Alumni Association assisted in the revision of its newsletter to ensure that college and faculty accomplishments were reported and a liaison officer was appointed to gather "newsworthy" items for submission to university public relations organizations.

Progress was slow but steady and then, as so often happens in strategic planning, unexpected intrusive factors forced a reordering of priorities. The National League for Nursing Accreditation Site Visit completed in spring, prior to the dean's arrival, was not fully successful, and the college was required to submit a two-year progress report addressing recommendations set forth regarding faculty and curriculum. The immediate need to engage in curriculum and program revision, to ensure that the accreditation status of the college would not remain in jeopardy, required intensive coordination of students, faculty and administration efforts. Needless to say, the National League Report did little to improve morale.

However, the dean came with a background that proved to be helpful in revising the curriculum for NLN approval. She willingly accessed

external consultants and shared her knowledge as the accreditation site visitor. This gave the faculty much needed direction. As a member of the NLN Board of Review, she was able to "shore up" student and faculty confidence. Ultimately, the Progress Report was well received by the National League for Nursing and the college was granted full accreditation. The dean and the faculty were elated with this accomplishment.

The work pertaining to the NLN Accreditation Progress Report was not yet completed when in the autumn quarter of 1979 the faculty of the university went on strike. Although the dean had worked in other institutions that had collective bargaining, she had never been involved in a strike, thus she was less than confident in her ability to respond appropriately. University administration declared that regular classes were to be maintained and college administrators were to monitor and record attendance. Dean Spero vividly recalled the day she naively turned to the College of Nursing and Health Administrative Committee, composed of two faculty representatives, six department chairs, three assistant deans and one assistant to the dean for help with the task and was advised by eight of the committee, who held memberships in the American Association of University Professors (AAUP), that it was an "administrative" problem and then proceeded to leave the room. She felt intense inner conflict when she had to "break the picket line" to enter Procter Hall or address students' and parents' inquiries regarding lost class and practice experience. The strike was orderly and once agreement was reached, faculty and students returned to resume activities directed toward goal achievement. Collective bargaining is now an established norm at the University of Cincinnati.

Having successfully negotiated National League for Nursing Accreditation and a faculty strike, Dean Spero resumed strategic planning. Faculty morale seemed to have improved, thus fiscal resources and faculty development became high priorities.

One of the strengths of the new dean that was critical to functioning successfully in her role was being able to manage monies allotted the school in a manner that enhanced the working of the college. In 1978, the operating budget of the college was a little over two million dollars, only 62 percent of which was from a General Funds

Left: Public health nurses' kit donated by Karen Byers (Class of 1975).

base. More than 68 percent of the graduate program operating budget was derived from "soft" money. As a result of previously mandated budget reductions, the college had been forced to depend upon the interest from endowments to support faculty salaries, and these were now significantly eroded. Heavy reliance on external funds and endowments for established programs placed the college at considerable risk of faculty reduction or program elimination at a time when student enrollment was increasing and community demand for new graduate programs was on the rise. Dean Spero believed that external funds should be acquired primarily for program innovation and developmental activities, rather than for the maintenance of faculty, primary educational activities and essential support systems. The halcyon days of big spending for higher education were on the wane and university budgets were becoming increasingly restricted, but the data were strong enough to approach university administration with a request for additional fiscal support. Negotiations with central administration were successful and it was agreed that upon termination of external grants personnel salaries would be replaced by General Funds to ensure program stabilization.

The infusion of General Funds was a temporary reprieve allowing faculty and administration to creatively pursue new avenues of support in order to achieve its growth objectives.

How the faculty perceives itself and how it believes it is perceived by others results in a synergism that may invoke latent energies for the purpose of moving in new directions. These same perceptions may impede progress and change. At the time of Dean Spero's arrival, it seemed that the faculty viewed themselves as "good teachers," and were rightfully proud of their graduates who were held in high esteem both locally and nationally. Although the faculty aspired to regain the national recognition that the college had held in the past, energies were primarily directed inward. There appeared to be little internal consistency in relation to faculty performance expectations; no clearly identified objectives for collective faculty development and no systematic way to award meritorious behaviors. The faculty subscribed to the norms of scholarship expected in academia, however they had restricted their energies to obtaining program grants for new program development to supplement the budget following the nine percent reduction that occurred in 1977.

In 1978, the faculty complement included nine doctorally prepared, 55 master's prepared and four baccalaureate prepared faculty. The National League for Nursing Accreditation Site Visit Report made imperative the need to increase the percentage of doctorally prepared faculty and to develop a workload plan to increase faculty scholarship activities. Administration support for developmental activities included (1) provision of academic and professional leaves; (2) financial support for faculty travel, attendance at professional meetings and continuing education workshops; (3) released time for scholastic activities and the provision of equipment and supplies to reduce the burdens associated with grant and research proposal development. An assistant dean of Research and Academic Development was appointed to coordinate the research efforts of the faculty. The dean also established two research accounts to provide "seed money" for student and faculty research. The faculty worked diligently to upgrade the criteria for appointment, promotion and

tenure as well as procedures for awarding merit. Tenured faculty who did not hold doctoral degrees were encouraged to enroll in graduate study. As there were limited state monies for salary increases, salary improvement was accomplished by the awarding of merit and equity adjustments.

Alumnus James Ruff ('76) entered the College of Nursing and Health upon returning from serving in Vietnam. At the college he was one of three men, but he was the only African-American male. It had been a long time since men had been students in the college: about a dozen were in the class of '77. Upon graduation Ruff continued working for Procter & Gamble, but now he was working as an occupational health nurse. He also became a member of the South West Ohio Association of Occupational Health Nurses.

"Yes, I remember two white males in the class of 1976. They were Ron Erb and Mike Masters. I do not remember the males in other classes," Ruff says. "I had a full-time job with Procter & Gamble. My age, gender and race were not as important as maintaining my job and completing the nursing program. I felt the range of reactions were normal. I had to focus on the goal. I do not recall blatant hostility. There were many people who were cordial, helpful and collegial."

When Ruff started at the College of Nursing, he had been one term short of a science degree, but because of the need to earn money he had dropped out of Knoxville College and enlisted in the Air Force.

"I felt that if I went to Vietnam and returned alive, the G.I. Bill education benefit would make college cost affordable," says Ruff.

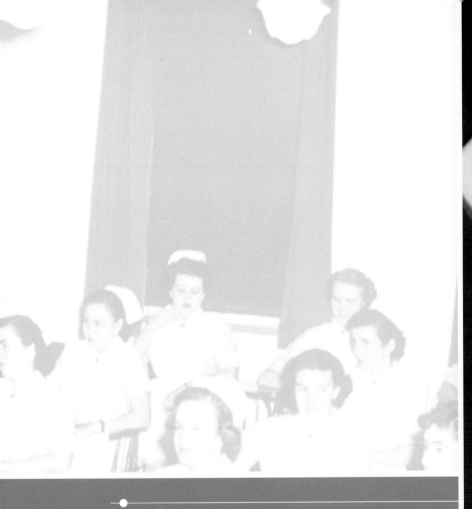

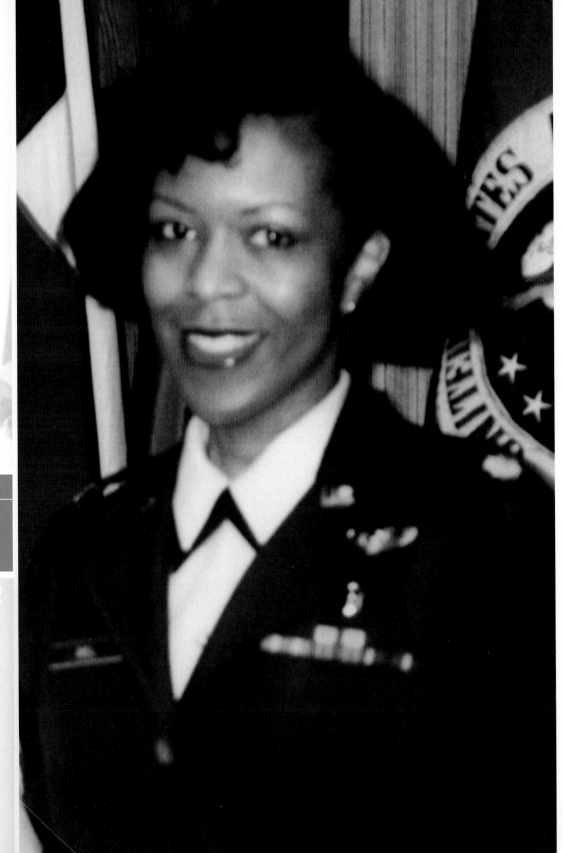

1970 • Four students are killed by Ohio National Guardsmen at Kent State University, starting a decade of unrest on college campuses for students and faculty alike.

1976 • Three men graduated: James Ruff, Ronald Erb, Michael Masters. They are not the first, but they are the first in "modern times."

EMBRACING TECHNOLOGY 1980–1989

Chapter Ten

10

In 1984, the college received the Ohio Regents Award for Excellence. Monies from this award combined with a grant from the Helene Fuld Foundation, a Computer-Based Information System grant and an Ohio Instructional Equipment Award were used to develop a sophisticated computer classroom and interactive video learning station. Faculty soon became involved in designing computer-assisted instruction models and other computer-related instruction technologies. The College of Nursing and Health was the first college on campus to produce an interactive video disc for instructional purposes.

In the '80s, the college became known as a center for gerontology nursing education, practice and research. The impetus to focus on this area of health care came as a result of a Robert Wood Johnson Teaching Nursing Home Project Award that was received in 1982. Faculty then could hold joint appointments in two area nursing homes and provide consultation to several other such facilities. The Continuing Education Program was designated as the Nursing Home Area Training Center, and in that capacity it provided educational programs for more than 1,000 individuals annually. The college became part of a consortium composed of the Schools of Nursing at the University of Oregon Health Science Center, Eugene, Oregon; SUNY–Binghamton; UCLA; and the University of Wisconsin–Madison to study incontinence in the elderly. The college engaged in funded collaborative research with the Cincinnati Center for Developmental Disorders and the colleges of Medicine and Pharmacy.

During Dean Spero's tenure, the number of faculty with earned doctorates increased from the original nine to 32 and by 1989, 62 per-

> "Most importantly, from this early ground-breaking interprofessional educational experience, we ended up with a stronger, more comprehensive approach to patient care and an appreciation for one another professionally."
> —Donna M. Fick, PhD, RN, FGSA, FAAN

Right: Class of 1983.

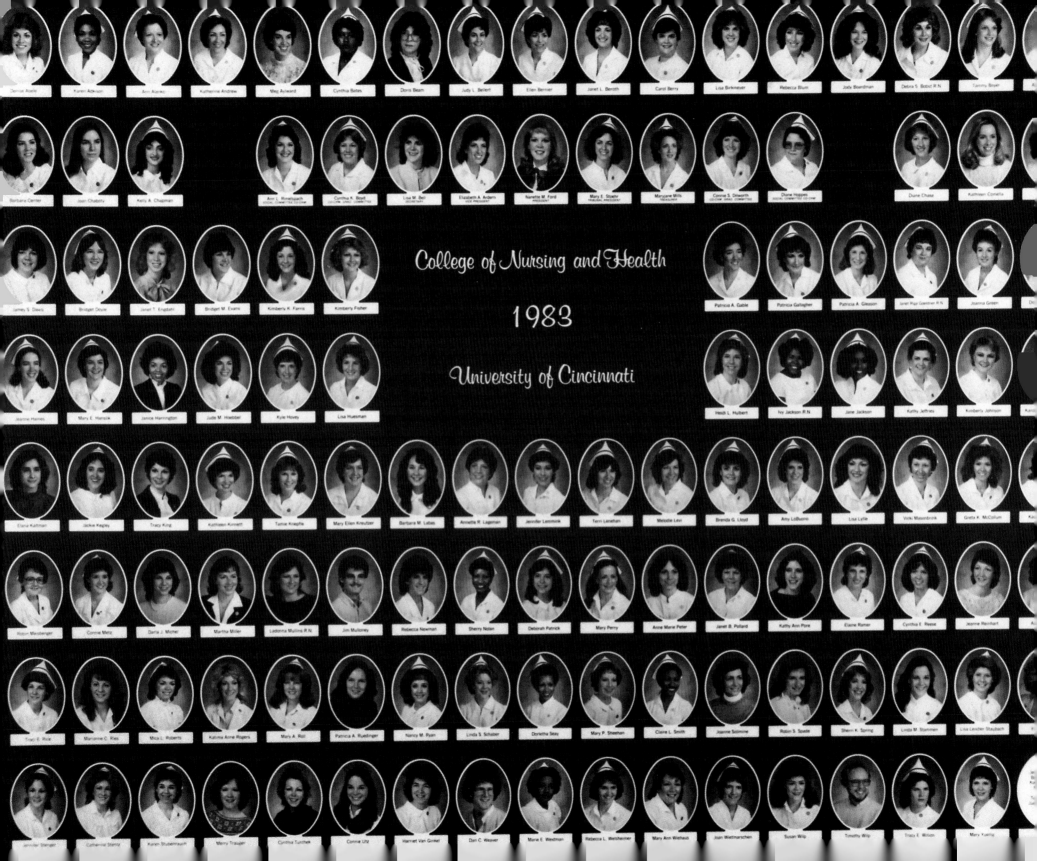

College of Nursing and Health

1983

University of Cincinnati

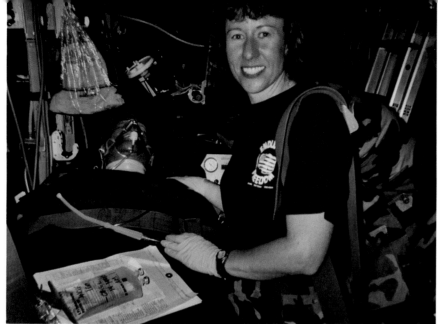

Top: U.S. Air Force Major Mary T. Schlaechter Carlisle (Class of 1988) served in the Critical Care Air Transport Team.

Right: Pictured from left to right: Margaret Duvall Baum, who wore the 1889 uniform worn by those first five "pupil nurses" enrolled in the Cincinnati Training School for Nurses, the forerunner of the UC College of Nursing and Health; Susan Pert Earley, '66, who wore an original 1895 uniform originally owned by Emma Lawrence Hofmann, '95; Patrice Steurenberg, '78, who modeled the "apron style" uniform, which appeared about 1909; Teresa Cox, '78, who modeled the 1922 uniform previously owned by Clara Gestel; Carolyn Hadley, '80, who wore the pink probationary uniform that was first introduced in 1914, was established in 1915 and last worn in 1932; Patti Spahr, '82, who modeled the probationary uniform worn in 1933, which featured a shawl collar rather than the traditional crisp white one. This introduced the "basic blue uniform:" Carol Bussey, '81, who displayed the standard uniform of students through 1970. Finally, three current students, who modeled the current uniform: Christine Wandell, Margo Weber and Chuck Washburn.

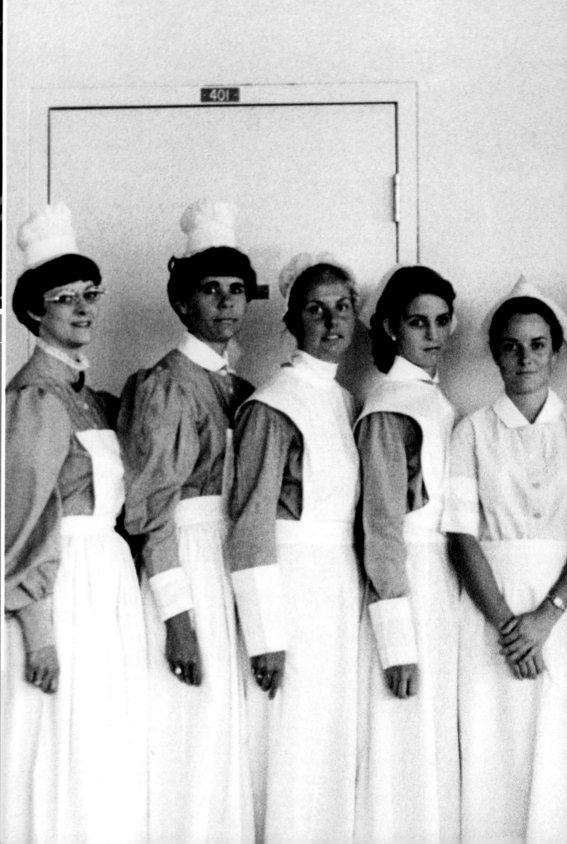

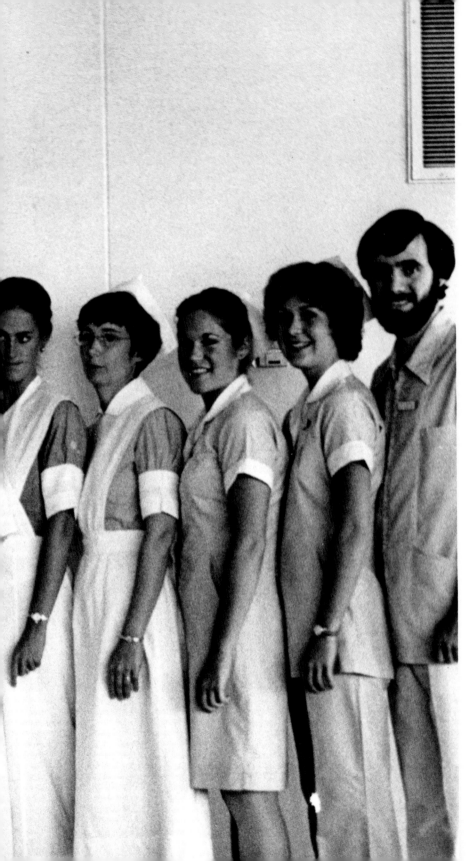

cent of the full-time faculty held doctorates. Scholarly publications increased and are frequently cited by others. During the 1988 fiscal year, the college received more than $280,000 in external research support and an additional $402,000 in programmatic grant and student stipend.

"In 1987, as a new student at the University of Cincinnati College of Nursing and Health, I was privileged to train under the mentorship of Ann McCracken, PhD, RNC, Evelyn Fitzwater, DSN, RN, and Gregg Warshaw, MD, and to be part of a Robert Wood Johnson (RWJ)–funded teaching nursing home project that began in the 1980s at Maple Knoll Village. This particular collaboration focused on a shared primary nursing model. As hoped by RWJ, the program influenced both the university and the nursing home staff and patients, but it also had a profound effect on me and other students who came through this collaboration and worked in Maple Knoll Village as our clinical site (McCracken-Knights, 1984).

"At the clinical site, we worked and trained side-by-side with other disciplines. We would visit the nursing home with medical, nutrition and pharmacy students. We would all assess the patient (usually together, if not overwhelming) and then come back to the conference room and discuss our experience, our assessment, and where we thought we could add value in improving care for this particular patient. Many times we would have different perspectives, but all were valued, and we had fun learning and caring for older adults together. Most importantly, from this early ground-breaking interprofessional educational experience, we ended up with a stronger, more comprehensive

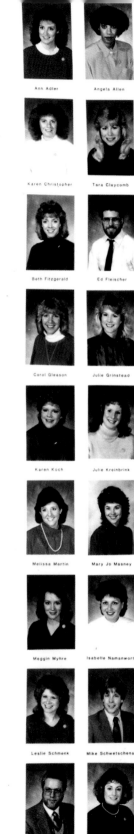

Ann Adler | Angela Allen | Kathleen Amstutz | Susan Atkinson | Barbara Baker | Julie Baumann | Nita Beebe | Cheryl Bigelow | Milissa Billingsley | Nancy Boeckman | Karen Boesherz | Lynette Boyers | Vicki Brown | Laura Brush | Lisa Cahoon | Kelly Christian

Karen Christopher | Tara Claycomb | Margaret Conaton | Latonya Croom | Mary Czinege | Lisa Dale | Shonna Day | Chris Dowling | Karen Ellis | Gail Enright | Regina Erpelding | Anne Etges | Jennifer Farwick | Cristina Fernandez | Beverly Fershtman | Kathryn Finkelstein

Beth Fitzgerald | Ed Fleischer | Jerry Schwartz, President | Nancy Brown, Vice-President | Beth Tarr, Treasurer | Barbara Doggett, Secretary | Barbara Simpson, Grad. Comm. Co-Chair. | Tammy Wilson, Grad. Comm. Co-Chair. | Teresa Herrmann, Fundraising Co-Chair. | Maribeth Thesing, Fundraising Co-Chair. | Marjorie McCarthy, Social Comm. Co-Chair. | Mary Eiser, Social Comm. Co-Chair. | Kim Fontana | Theresa Gaughan

University of Cincinnati
College of
Nursing and Health
1987

Carol Gleason | Julie Grinstead | Tamara Hartsell | Audrey Henley | Therese Holden | | Noreen Huber | Antoinette Jenkins | Theresa Johnson | Cheryl Kaminsky | Linda Kern

Karen Koch | Julie Kreinbrink | Gigi Landom | Roseann Larkins | Kay Larson | | Kathy Lauer | Jennifer Logan | Cindy Luca | Irene Margolin | Susan Marketos

Melissa Martin | Mary Jo Masney | Angie Matacia | Shelley Mather | Yvonne Maynard | | Janet McGinnis | Colleen McMahon | Jody Miller | James Millward | Jemela Murib

Meggin Myhre | Isabelle Namanworth | Andi Niemann | Deborah O'Hanian | Judith Paat | Jennifer Pieper | Elaine Plummer | Lisa Pollard | Kathryn P'Simer | Jean Rasfeld | Diane Reed | Debra Riedinger | Don Robinson | Mary Roll | Mary Ryan | Monica Saleh

Leslie Schmenk | Mike Schwetschenau | Sheila Sferra | Janine Sidey | Myra Simmons | Sandra Sites | Deborah Smith | Michelle Smith | Susan Smith | Debra Soete | Lisa Steinhaus | Susan Stoffregen | Marina Svetlik | Laura Sweeney | Amy Szczesny | Joann Szeto

Mike Terrana | Lenna Toleski | Joanne Turner | Sharon Ungar | Michelle Vielhauer | Karen Wagner | Sheri Waked | Mary Walker | Ann Wechter | Wendy Weisberg | Angela Weitzel | Rebecca White | Melissa Wilson | Brenda Worcester | Veronica Zierden

approach to patient care and an appreciation for one another pro-fessionally."— Donna M. Fick, PhD, RN, FGSA, FAAN, The Pennsylvania State University College of Nursing, "What I Know For Sure: The Value of Interprofessional Education and Practice in Geriatrics and an Exciting New Collaboration for Our Journal," *Journal of Gerontological Nursing,* June 2014, Volume 40 · Issue 6: 3-4

1982 • The college was one of only 11 schools of nursing nationally to receive the prestigious Robert Wood Johnson Teaching Nursing Home Project Grant for a full-year funding period. The site of implementation was Maple Knoll Village. As a result of this project, the following year the College of Nursing was designated a "Nursing Home Training Center" by the Ohio Department of Health.

1984 • The college received the Ohio Board of Regents Executive Award to establish computer-assisted instruction for undergraduate students. A subsequent grant from the Helene Fuld Health Trust in 1986 made it possible to complete the computer classroom and laboratory.

1986 • The college received Advanced Nurse Training Grant awards from the Department of Health and Human Services, Division of Nursing, to implement master's curricula in Oncology Nursing (1986) and Gerontological Nursing (1988). The college also received the Area Health Education Center Special Initiative Award to establish an educational network for professional nurses employed in caring for the elderly.

1987 • The College of Nursing received the Ross Laboratories Award for "Leadership in Long Term Care." The college became one of 15 institutions chosen by IBM to develop computer-assisted interactive video for health sciences.

Left: Class of 1987.

ANSWERING THE CALL 1990–1999
Chapter Eleven

11

Carolyn Nicholson entered the nurse anesthesia program as a student in October 1970 and graduated after 18 months with a diploma in April 1972. Then she went back and got her BS in education from UC ('86). She remained as faculty and taught clinically as well as didactically within the Department of Anesthesia in the College of Medicine.

Then in 1991 the Nurse Anesthesia Program came under the College of Nursing. "I saw a lot of changes in the way we taught," she says.

In 1945 when the program was founded, most programs were six months in duration because not many forms of anesthesia were available so there was not much to teach. Then as medicine advanced, there were more things to teach, but most of it was clinical as opposed to didactic. The developments weren't necessarily in higher education.

"You observed CRNAs before you taught and tried to improve upon it. We did not have as many resources available to us and it was not always easy to access teaching materials." The presentations were made using an overhead projector. "Initially I considered the overhead projector to be really neat but it was not long before it became obsolete!"

"When we progressed from the overhead to using slides, we made our own slides. If I wanted a color slide then I had to hand paint them. Otherwise, it was black letters on a white background. Then we got blue backgrounds with white letters!"

"Then the university had an AV department and we, as faculty, were allotted a certain amount in the budget to have slides made, but it was very expensive. If you wanted to add a photo, you had to have it scanned. Now—we can get photos and access to articles. Just pull up a PDF and stick it right in there! It's so much easier to access. Back when I started, the amount of time to prepare lectures was incredible: it took hundreds of hours."

"Textbooks were expensive then—of course, they're still expensive—but there was no electronic access like today."

"I have to say the technology has not necessarily made students smarter or more prepared. In the past, students read the material ahead of time and we'd discuss it. Today's technology makes it easier for the instructor to prepare lectures and perhaps more entertaining for the student. Maybe now there's more of an expectation of 'just tell me what I need to know.'"

Carolyn Nicholson started in nurse anesthesia as an 18-month diploma student and ended up working there for 42 years: "It was a wonderful career."

"In 1945, nurse anesthesia consisted primarily of open drop ether, spinals and nitrous oxide/oxygen inhalation. Around World War II thiopental became available [Sodium thiopental, given by injection, took seconds to affect the patient and was just what they needed in a war context.] The inhalation and intravenous agents used today were unavailable at that time."

Nurse Anesthesia Program Director and Assistant Professor of Clinical William Terry Ray, PhD, MNSc, CRNA, congratulates Carolyn Nicholson, CRNA, at her retirement celebration.

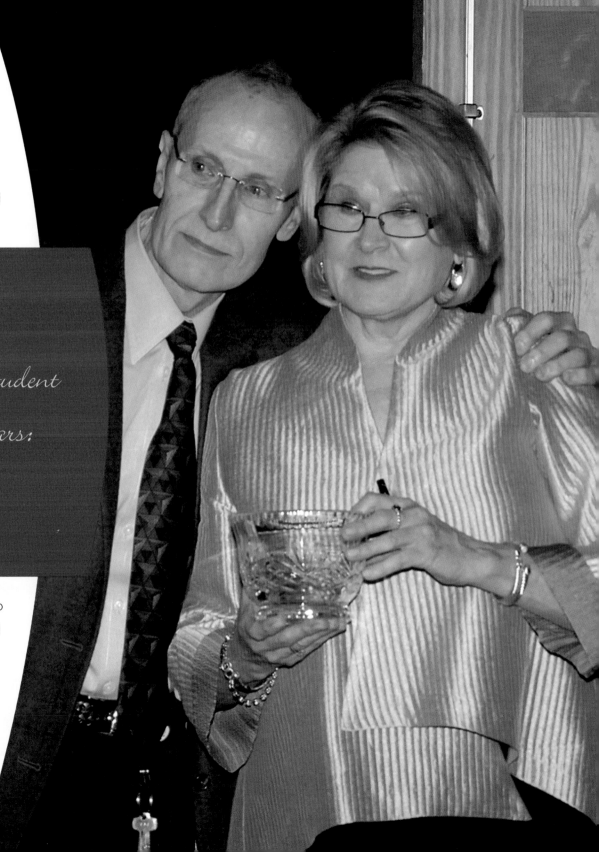

"In 1846 was the first public demonstration of anesthetics at Massachusetts General Hospital. It would take the next 50 years for the nurses a natural skill for caring for the patient. And it was a low-paying job and nurses were willing to work for low wages."

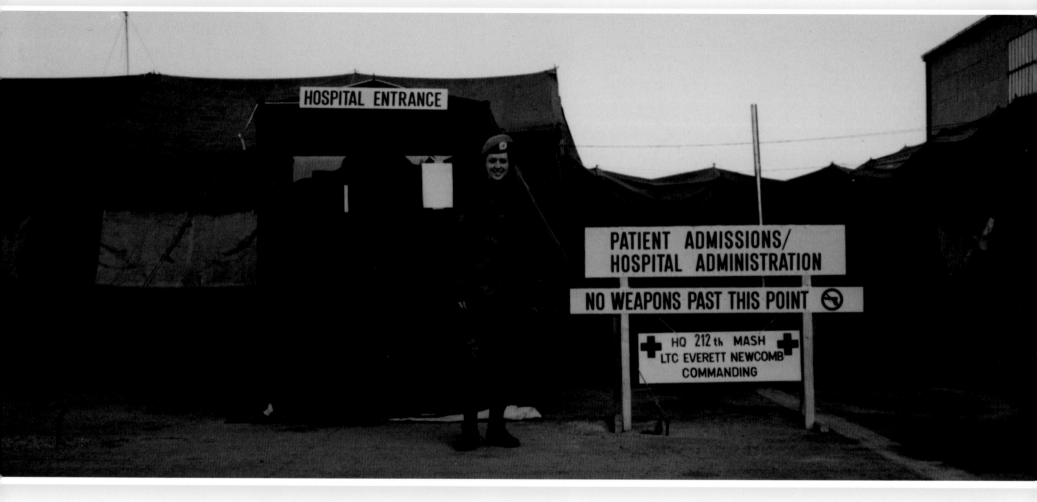

anesthesia to be considered safe since often it was administered by untrained people (medical students, surgical assistants and even family members). Although surgeons called upon their colleagues to assume the role of the anesthesia provider, most physicians considered it not their job—their job was to operate. The solution for the surgeons was to train the nurses and to train them well. They saw in So the nurses were the first group to answer the call. In the 1900s nurse anesthesia began to flourish. Famous surgeon Charles Mayo had his own private anesthetist, Alice Magaw. Magaw was very skilled at open drop ether, where gauze would be placed by the patient's mouth, and ether (or an ether-chloroform mix) was dropped on the gauze. Providing a safe anesthetic for the patient and allowing a

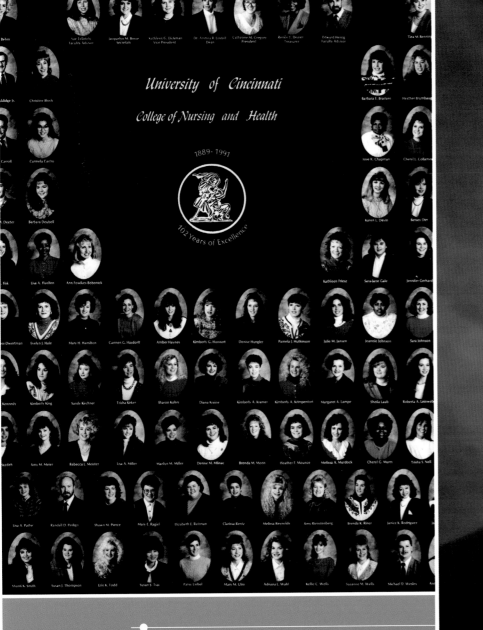

University of Cincinnati

College of Nursing and Health

1889-1991

102 Years of Excellence

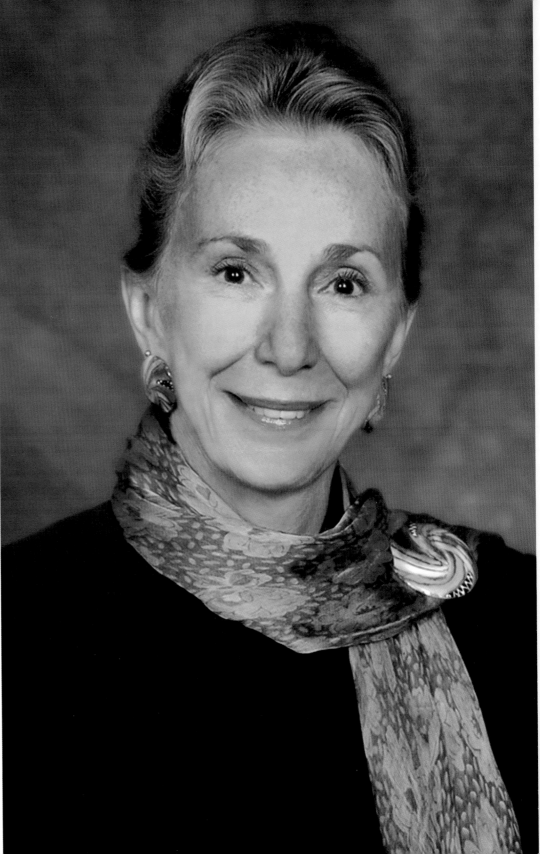

Top: Class of 1991.
Left: Alumna Theresa A. Floegel served in the U.S. Army Nurse Corps from 1990–1995. This photo is from her deployment in 1992–1993 with the 212th MASH in support of the United Nations peacekeeping forces in Croatia.
Right: Dean Andrea Lindell

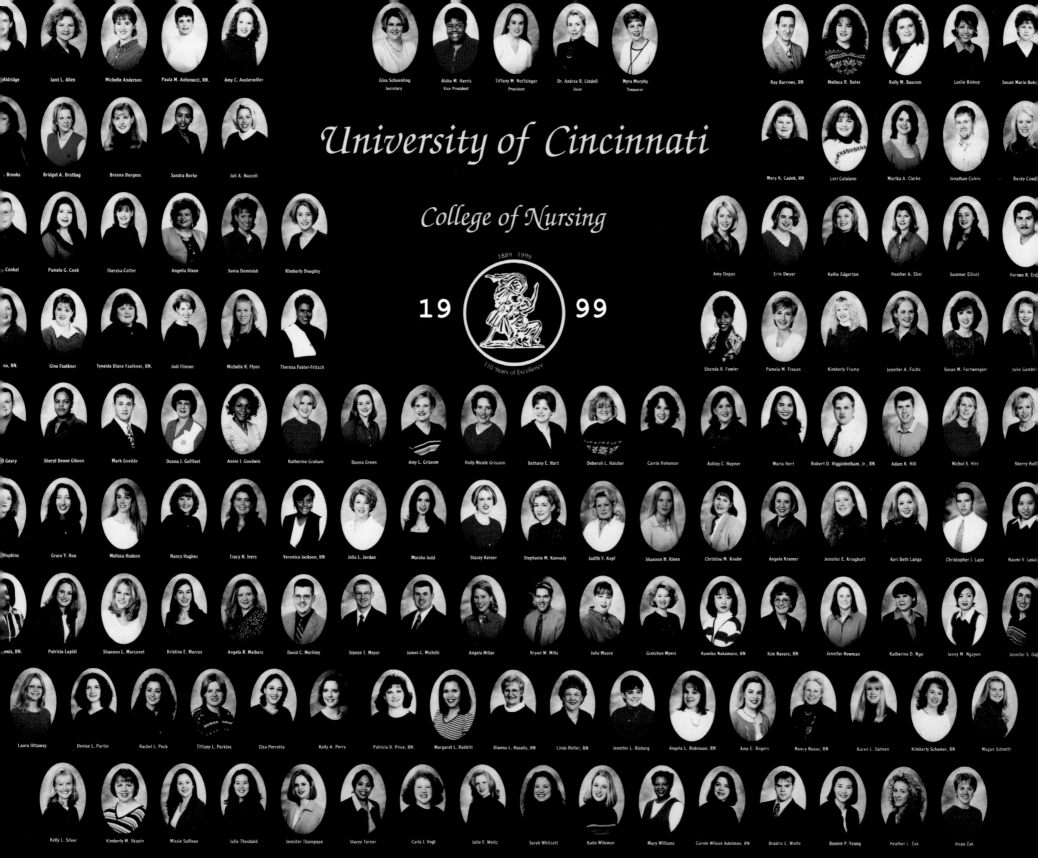

University of Cincinnati

College of Nursing

1889 1999

19 99

110 Years of Excellence

Aldridge · Jami L. Allen · Michelle Anderson · Paula M. Antonucci, RN. · Amy C. Austermiller

Gina Schoenling
Secretary

Aisha M. Harris
Vice President

Tiffany M. Noftsinger
President

Dr. Andrea R. Lindell
Dean

Myra Murphy
Treasurer

Ray Barrows, RN · Melissa R. Bates · Kelly M. Baucom · Leslie Bishop · Susan Marie Bohi

Brooks · Bridget A. Brothag · Brenna Burgess · Sandra Burke · Juli A. Buzzeli

Mary K. Cadek, RN · Lori Catalano · Marika A. Clarke · Jonathan Colvin · Becky Coodl

Conkel · Pamela G. Cook · Theresa Cotter · Angelia Dixon · Sonia Dominish · Kimberly Doughty

Amy Dupps · Erin Dwyer · Kellie Edgerton · Heather A. Ehni · Summer Elliott · Herman R. Era

na, RN. · Gina Faulkner · Tyneida Diane Faulkner, RN. · Jodi Flinner · Michelle R. Flynn · Theresa Foster-Fritsch

Shonda R. Fowler · Pamela M. Freson · Kimberly Frump · Jennifer A. Fuchs · Susan M. Furtwengler · Julie Gambil

Geary · Sheryl Denee Gibson · Mark Goedde · Donna J. Goffinet · Annie J. Goodwin · Katherine Graham · Donna Green · Amy L. Grissom · Holly Nicole Grissom · Bethany E. Hart · Deborah L. Hatcher · Carrie Heheman · Ashley C. Hepner · Maria Hert · Robert D. Higginbotham, Jr., RN · Adam K. Hill · Nichol S. Hirz · Sherry Hoff

Hopkins · Grace Y. Hou · Melissa Hudson · Nancy Hughes · Tracy N. Ivers · Veronica Jackson, RN · Julia L. Jordan · Marsha Judd · Stacey Keiner · Stephanie M. Kennedy · Judith Y. Kepf · Shannon N. Kleen · Christina M. Knabe · Angela Kramer · Jennifer E. Krieghoff · Keri Beth Lange · Christopher J. Lape · Naomi V. Lesch

ewis, RN. · Patricia Lupidi · Shannon L. Marconet · Kristina E. Marcus · Angela R. Meibers · David C. Merhley · Steven T. Meyer · James C. Michels · Angela Miller · Bryan W. Mills · Julie Moore · Gretchen Myers · Kumiko Nakamura, RN · Kim Navaro, RN · Jennifer Newman · Katherine D. Ngo · Jenny M. Nguyen · Jennifer S. Oa

Laura Ottaway · Denise L. Partin · Rachel L. Peck · Tiffany L. Perkins · Elsa Perrotta · Kelly A. Perry · Patricia D. Price, RN. · Margaret L. Rabbitt · Dianna L. Rasulis, RN · Linda Reiter, RN · Jennifer L. Risberg · Angela L. Robinson, RN · Amy C. Rogers · Nancy Russo, RN · Karen L. Salmen · Kimberly Schamer, RN · Megan Schmitt

Kelly L. Silver · Kimberly M. Skapin · Missie Sullivan · Julie Theobald · Jennifer Thompson · Stacey Turner · Carla J. Vogt · Julie F. Weitz · Sarah Whitsett · Katie Wilemon · Mary Williams · Carole Wilson Adelman, RN · Bradric C. Wolfe · Bonnie P. Yeung · Heather L. Zak · Hope Zak

surgeon to have optimal operating conditions required an incredible amount of technical and observational skills.

"Magaw not only administered anesthesia but she kept track of the anesthetics she administered and noted her observations and effects of anesthesia upon her patients. This culminated with her famous publication in 1906 describing the administration of over 14,000 anesthetics without an associated anesthetic death. The first formalized nurse anesthetist programs were from 1909–1914. Soon after they began more formalized programs. One of the most famous nurse anesthesia programs was Lakeside School of Nurse Anesthesia in Cleveland, OH founded by Agatha Hodgins in 1915. Agatha Hodgins was the founder of the professional organization known today as the American Association of Nurse Anesthetists (AANA)."

Contributions by nurses to the war efforts in both WWI and WWII had a huge impact on the growth of nurse anesthesia programs. Initially most programs were hospital based, but later a college association or affiliation was encouraged. The first time a qualifying exam was required was in 1945. Criteria were established for accreditation by the AANA in 1952. There was a rebound in the 60s for nurse-anesthesia programs and applicants, but the AANA maintained it was vital to have fewer programs with better educational standards.

"In the 70s and 80s, the AANA encouraged those of us who were teaching to get advanced degrees, so I obtained a master's degree in education in 1986. Our program came under the College of Nursing in '91 and today it is moving toward the doctoral level."

Many of the program's graduates have played important roles in the field. For example, Wanda Wilson is the current executive director of the AANA. Founder of UC College of Nursing's nurse anesthesia program, Mary Alice Costello, and graduates Peggy McFadden and Wanda Wilson have served in the capacity of president of the AANA. The program has had the distinction of having four individuals awarded the Alice Magaw Outstanding Clinical Practitioner award: Jeanne Coffey, Sarah T. Johnson, Elaine Klein and Carolyn Nicholson. And Vera Griner was awarded the Program Director of the year.

"The earliest programs realized the importance of education and set the program standards for themselves. UC is one of the oldest and most reputable programs still in existence today. You start out and you continue to perfect it. We did a great job with what

Left: Class of 1999.
Right: This bust of Florence Nightingale was given to the college in 1996 by Joan Nightingale Fox, the great-grandniece of Florence Nightingale. The college was modeled on the Nightingale Training School for Nurses in London.

we had. We answered the call; we had foresight; and we continue to grow," she says. Just like a commercial of the 90s, she adds, "We've come a long way, baby!"

In the beginning, operations only took place to amputate or for fractures: no surgery unless absolutely necessary.

"It's been a phenomenal career. I've had a great career. It's amazing all the opportunities I've had. It was a great job and a very rewarding opportunity to know that I have helped teach nearly 700 students in my career."

"If you've had an anesthetic in Cincinnati, most likely it is a nurse anesthetist who graduated from our programs. It's really been a privilege to have had this opportunity."

"In the beginning, operations only took place to amputate or for fractures: no surgery unless absolutely necessary. Then ether came along and the first public demonstration of it clearly changed things. But it took a long time for anesthesia to be accepted by the public. It took for someone to be qualified and it took a nurse to answer the call. Nurses took it upon themselves to establish an education requirement and guidelines, and to keep improving themselves and raising the standards."

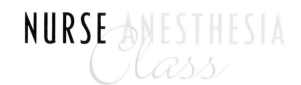

NURSE ANESTHESIA Class

Nurse anesthetists have been providing anesthesia care to patients in the United States for 150 years. As one of the oldest existing educational programs for nurse anesthetists, the University of Cincinnati Nurse Anesthesia program has a long history of academic and clinical excellence.

Certified Registered Nurse Anesthetists (CRNAs) are advanced practice nurses and anesthesia professionals who safely administer approximately 32 million anesthetics each year in the United States. CRNAs provide anesthesia care to patients before, during and after surgery or childbirth. CRNAs practice with a high degree of autonomy as they work collaboratively with other health care providers such as surgeons, anesthesiologists, dentists and podiatrists.

The UC Nurse Anesthesia program requires 28 months (seven semesters) of full-time study. Clinical experience begins in the first semester to allow students to integrate and apply concepts learned in the classroom.

Effective January 2016, the program will transition to a BSN to DNP program pending approval by the Council on Accreditation.

1990 ● The college received a second Helene Fuld Health Trust grant to further develop computer-assisted learning. The doctoral program (PhD) in nursing was implemented. The Nursing Faculty Development for Substance Abuse Program was introduced. The Center for Nursing Research, co-sponsored by the College of Nursing and University Hospital Patient Care Services, was established in 1990.

1992 ● The "on site" Center for Nursing Research facility was accomplished in 1992. The college also established a joint master's degree with the (then) College of Business Administration to award the MSN/MBA dual degrees.

1993 ● UC's College of Nursing and Health was one of three universities in Ohio selected to participate in the Advance Practice Pilot Program. The college was among the first to offer an Accelerated Pathway program that allows non-nursing degree holders to quickly become an RN and earn the MSN degree.

1994 ● The college established a health initiative with Project Succeed within the Cincinnati Public School system. The college became an affiliate of George Mason University's World Health Organization collaborating site.

1995 ● Due to phenomenal productivity, the Center for Nursing Research was officially named the Institute for Nursing Research in 1995. Under the aegis of the Institute are the Center for Gerontological Nursing Excellence (GNE) and the Center for Addiction Research (CAR). The college established the corporation for Nurses in Advanced Practice, Inc. (NIAP), a corporation of the College of Nursing. It was founded to provide nursing services on a contractual basis. One entity under this corporation is the Health Resource Center, located in the Free Store/Foodbank. The center is staffed by faculty and students, who see as many as 200 indigent clients each month.

1998 ● The College of Allied Health Sciences became the university's 16th college (at the time), separating from what is now known as the College of Nursing.

WELCOMING A NEW MILLENNIUM 2000–2009

Chapter Twelve

12

Children often have dreams of what they want to be when they grow up. Many health care professionals can tell stories of how they fixed their teddy bears and dolls when they were "sick" or checked their friend's heart rate with plastic stethoscopes.

Andrea Lindell, PhD, an internationally respected nursing leader, isn't one of them.

Lindell wanted to enroll in a flight attendant school in New York City after graduating high school in her small Pennsylvania town, but the tuition was more than her parents could afford.

A friend attending a diploma hospital nursing program told Lindell that her three years tuition was less than half of the cost for one year at flight attendant school. It was a price Lindell's parents could afford, so she enrolled in the program—a decision that paved the way for a distinguished nursing career.

Lindell, dean of the College of Nursing, had been a pioneer in nursing education for more than 30 years. Her dedication

and commitment to advancing the field of nursing locally, nationally and internationally was honored by the National League for Nursing (NLN), which inducted her into its inaugural fellows class in 2007.

Fellows were selected by the NLN board of governors for their sustained and significant contributions to the field of nursing education, with the expectation that they serve as role models for those in the nursing profession.

"I love what I do," said Lindell. "I enjoy working with my team, sharing my expertise and mentoring leaders to continue moving nursing education forward."

Lindell's nursing career began in a hospital but quickly moved to education. After earning a bachelor's degree in nursing from Villa Maria College, she earned a master's in nursing and a doctorate from Catholic University of America.

Her initial focus was on psychiatric mental health, which she began teaching to nursing students at Catholic. While educating future

Right: Class of 2002.

University of Cincinnati

College of Nursing and Health

20 02

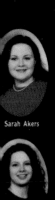
Sarah Akers

Daniel M. Albertz

Jennifer Amburgey

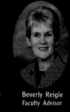
Tiffany N. Johnson
Secretary

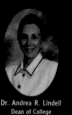
Mandi Barcikowski
President

Judy Laver
Faculty Advisor

Dr. Andrea R. Lindell
Dean of College

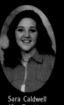
Beverly Reigle
Faculty Advisor

Sara Caldwell
Vice President

Julia Lutkenhoff
Treasurer

Katie Ankenbauer

Jennifer R. Ballman

Kimberly K. Bayl

mily W. Blanton

Kathryn Brosch

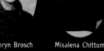
Misalena Chittum

Melissa Lynn Coby

Zakiya Copeland

Lisa Craig

Stephanie R. Davidson

Lisa R. Downto

Donna Dykes

Pam El-Hajj

Kristin A. Elliot

Rhonda Ellison

Peggy L. Ernst

Kimberlee Flannery

Lauren Flenner

Julie Froeliche

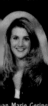
an Marie Gering

Jamie Rae Germann

Deidre Lynn Gillespie

Elizabeth Golder

Molly M. Grooms

Kelly C. Hannon

Keith Aric Harnist

Connie Hein

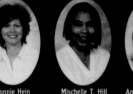
Mischelle T. Hill

Andrea J. Hinkst

Amy Hoffman

Melissa Ann Hunley

Laurie K. Karr

Liesl N. Kientz

Angela K. Kieviet

Rachel Koehler

Olivia Lally

Molly Lameier

Kimi Larson

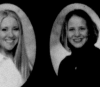
Jenni Limbert

Jennifer Loebker

Julia M. Lupidi

Lisa McQueen

Natalie Mirosh

Ginger Mohr

Roxana Moses

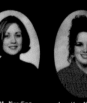
Amanda Muennich

Amanda Mullikin

Joy M. Neading

Jennifer Newport

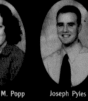
Amy Papania

Samantha M. Popp

Joseph Pyles

Amy Radcliff

Amanda M. Retzler

Jill L. Ritzi

Katie Schock

Tina Sicurella

Michael Edward Stacey

Donna Sue Sulli

S. Sunderhaus

Jennifer L. Taylor

McKenya Tessmer

Geraldine Tumenta

Kelly J. Vogler

Stephanie L. Voils

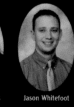
Erica Walker

Amanda Webb

Hannah R. Wells

Jason Whitefoot

Lisa A. Wietmarschen

Billita Williams

Megan Williams

Kertrice T. Wilson

Jen Wylie

nurses about their role in psychiatric mental health, Lindell then became interested in nursing administration.

She continued, "I firmly believe what the faculty and I do has a significant influence on the future of nursing education. We're training

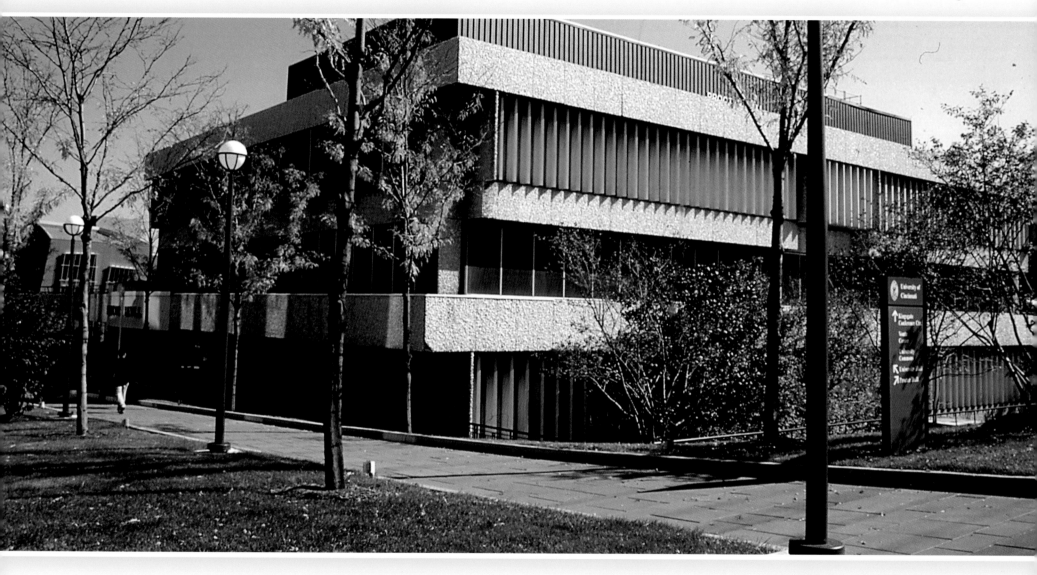

"I really enjoy being the facilitator and working with faculty and staff to enhance the quality and programs offered to nursing students," Lindell said.

students to provide exceptional health care to patients, as well as training those who will become nursing leaders and educators."

The former exterior of Procter Hall.

Lindell's administrative career began in 1975 as the director of the nursing graduate program at Catholic. She was there for two years before joining the nursing faculty at the University of New Hampshire.

In 1990, Lindell came to UC as dean and professor for the College of Nursing and Health. She was also named the associate senior vice president for academic affairs for the Academic Health Center.

Lindell's accomplishments during her 20 years at UC were extensive and include moving from a hospital-based nurse anesthesia program to a master's program; implementing a doctorate program; and developing new graduate-level practitioner programs such as neonatal, critical care, midwifery and genetics.

She also established a board of advisors to the college composed of community, corporate and health care leaders, and developed and fostered corporate partnerships on joint programs, research and professional development. The first board consisted of the following:

- R. L. Alhbrand
- Mary Ellen Betz
- J. Joseph Bonner
- Philip Barach
- Susan Jensen Brown
- Joseph Campanella
- Phillip Cox
- Lois Doyle
- Richard Fleming
- Oliver Gale
- Warren Haug
- Sandra Laney
- Kevin O'Brien
- Janet B. Rosen
- Frances Schloss
- O. Wayne Schneider
- Gerald Von Deylen
- Eric B. Yeiser
- Cynthia White
- Andrea Wiot

Lindell's passion for advancing nursing education and expertise in curriculum and instructional design, organizational management and behavior, fiscal analysis and management led to international partnerships in South Korea, Japan, China, Honduras, Mexico, Egypt and Jordan.

Her involvement and leadership with nursing committees and organizations included being past president of the American Association of Colleges of Nursing. What drove Lindell is simple. She loved what she was doing and wanted to keep moving nursing education forward.

"I like to go home every day and be happy about one thing I've accomplished," Lindell said. "Even if it's as simple as saying 'hello' to someone on my team that I haven't spoken with in a while. "Even the small things are important in our everyday life as we look to maintain quality," says Lindell.

COLLEGE OF NURSING
SUCCESSFUL IN RESEARCH
funding

In the early 1990s, the College of Nursing and Health became serious about nursing research. As a profession, nursing had been moving from the bedside to the research bench in a growing trend to nursing-oriented science.

Nurses were not only at the forefront of delivering quality health care. They were also playing an increasingly important part in developing it. In 1992, Lindell recruited Carol Deets, EdD, RN, as the college's associate dean for research. In addition, she would serve as director of the Center for Nursing Research, which was being developed at the time.

As the center grew, it was renamed in 1996 to the Institute for Nursing Research. Marilyn (Lynn) Sommers, PhD, RN, joined the center as the associate director. She later led the center as director and ultimately associate dean for nursing research until her transition to emeriti in 2006.

Where once any nurse "doing research" was at best a project director implementing someone else's protocol, today's nurse scientist is very likely to be the funded principal investigator directing a team of physicians or PhDs.

"In some areas nurses are now the senior mentoring scientist, and that's a real switch," said Sommers. By 2004, the college had achieved $1.8 million in research funding. Sommers, herself headed two major studies funded by the Centers for Disease Control and Prevention (CDC) and the National Institutes of Health (NIH).

The institute expanded further in 2008 and was renamed the Institute for Nursing Research and Scholarship to reflect the support provided for the scholarly work of faculty members.

In 2009, the College of Nursing had more than $1 million in research funding, had submitted 18 extramural grant proposals in the last six months of the year and had a strong presence in national nursing publications—all under the dynamic leadership of Dean Andrea Lindell, PhD.

"That leadership and the support for nursing research in the College of Nursing," said Cynthia Loveland Cook, PhD, is what drew her attention to UC and to her recently appointed position as associate dean of research.

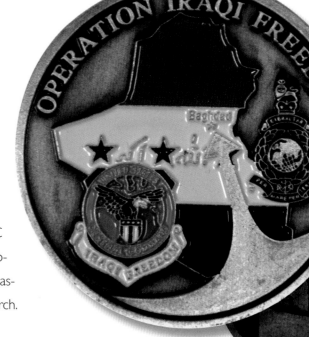

Iraqi Freedom Coin front and back.

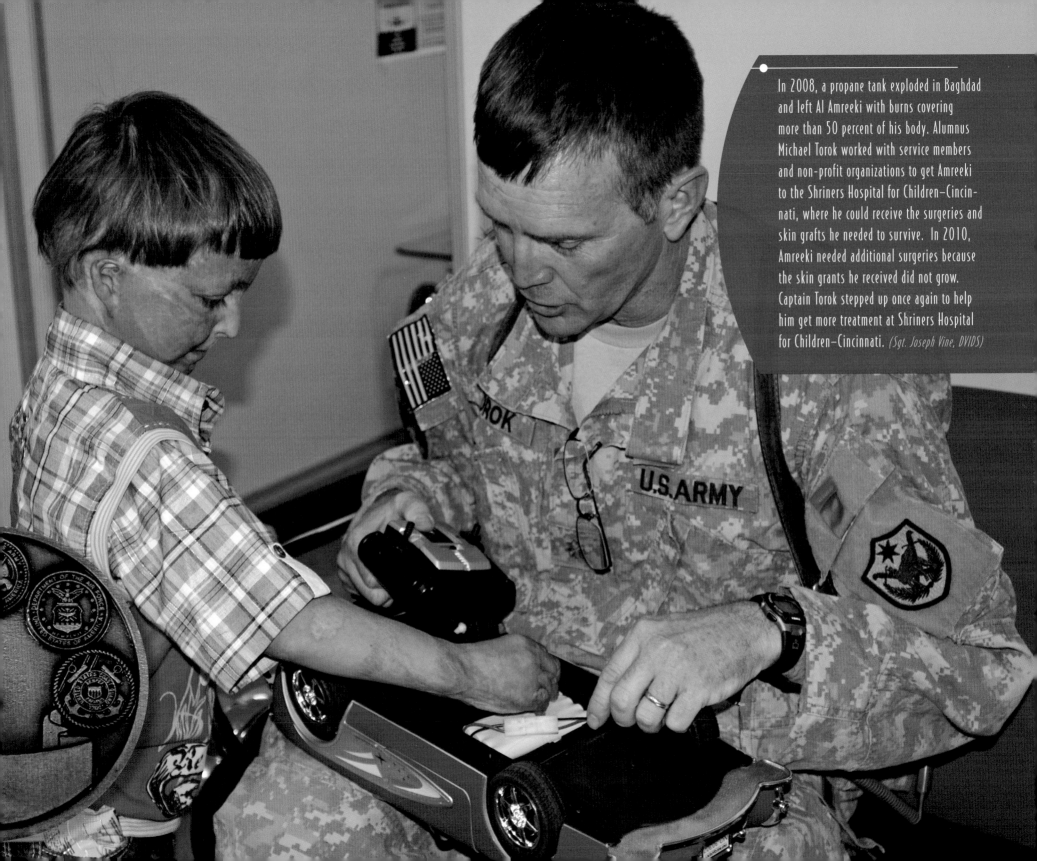

In 2008, a propane tank exploded in Baghdad and left Al Amreeki with burns covering more than 50 percent of his body. Alumnus Michael Torok worked with service members and non-profit organizations to get Amreeki to the Shriners Hospital for Children–Cincinnati, where he could receive the surgeries and skin grafts he needed to survive. In 2010, Amreeki needed additional surgeries because the skin grants he received did not grow. Captain Torok stepped up once again to help him get more treatment at Shriners Hospital for Children–Cincinnati. (Sgt. Joseph Vine, DVIDS)

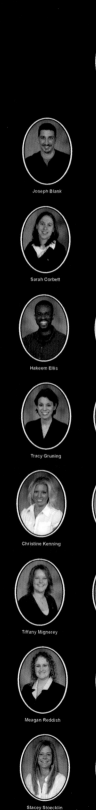
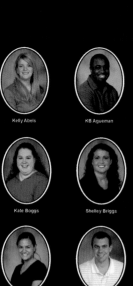
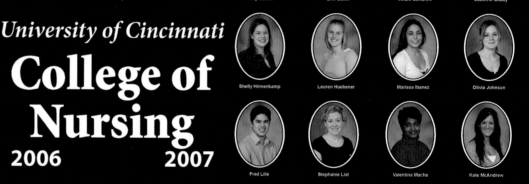

Kelly Abels

KB Agueman

Mark Ogg
President

Beth Purcell
Vice President

Andrea Lindell
Dean

Megan Schweller
Secretary

Sasha Simmons
Treasurer

Umaru Bah

Rebecca Baker

Joseph Blank

Kate Boggs

Shelley Briggs

Jamie Brown

Sarah Bunch

Amanda Busch

Erin Butt

Abby Cacini

Maria Caldwell

Jesy Clements

Tara Collett

Laura Conley

Della Conn

Sarah Corbett

Denise Costa

Cory Davis

Tameka Davis

Michael Domiano

Amanda Downing

Erika Drake

Jessica Drees

Jennifer Duggins

Lindsay Duncan

Brittney Duval

Suzanne Ehlers

Delores Ekuibe

Hakeem Ellis

Megan Elmendorf

Denise England

Megan Espersen

Amanda Fishman

Kelly Friesz

Christina Fugman

Bethelhem Gared

Amy Garlick

Erin Gatch

Tiffani Gendrew

Cathrine Gilday

Kristy Grimm

Tracy Gruning

Golda Gyabaa

Lori Harris

Jacqueline Henson

Nichloas Herrick

University of Cincinnati
College of
Nursing
2006   2007

Shelly Hinnenkamp

Lauren Huebener

Marissa Ibanez

Olivia Johnson

Kalpana Jyengar

Christine Kenning

Jessica Lamping

Suzanne Lee

Katie Lewis

Erika Lilie

Fred Lilie

Stephanie List

Valentina Macha

Kate McAndrew

Kourtney Merriweather

Tiffany Mignerey

Ellie Miller

Jessica Moon

Alyssa Murphy

Kristin Myers

Julie Nguyen

Joycelyn O'Connell

Erin O'Hara

Shannon Osterfeld

Tonia Owens

Lauren Piontek

Karla Prenger

Sally Raber

Meagan Reddish

Heidi Reder

Edie Ritzi

Diana Rogalski

Danielle Sallee

Stacy Samano

Heather Schmarr

Sarah Schmudde

Kelly Schomaker

Emily Serger

Carolyn Smith

Willam Snapp

Rob Stamper

Stacey Stoecklin

Crystal Straight

Antoinette Thomas

Robert Vandivier

Robert Weitzel

Erin Whitaker

Katie Widrig

Kristi Wieland

Sara Wimmer

Nicole Wise

Emily Wolff

Jodie Yee

Jennifer Zentner

"The faculty here are engaged in exciting research that will have an important impact locally and nationally," Cook said of current research studies on topics such as violence against providers in emergency departments, religiosity in adult transitions, nursing education, health behaviors, substance abuse, homelessness and health disparities.

And with the College of Nursing so close in proximity to other colleges within UC's Academic Health Center, "it becomes a wonderful setting for interdisciplinary research," she said.

ACADEMIC

During the 2000s, the college saw tremendous growth in enrollment. As graduate programs expanded and distance learning programs were offered, the reach of the college's educational programs expanded greatly. For the majority of the decade, these programs were led by Deets, who had become associate dean for Graduate Studies; and Lou Ann Emerson, DNSc, RN, who began her tenure with the college as an instructor in 1965 and retired as senior associate dean. In 2007, Madeleine (Mimi) T. Martin, EdD, RN, stepped into the role of associate dean for Undergraduate Programs following her tenure, which began in 1980.

Given the expansion, the Office of Student Affairs and the Center for Academic Technologies and Educational Resources (CATER) became further established to meet the increased needs of the growing number of students and the evolution of technology in nursing education. These departments continue to be critical partners in allowing the college to provide innovative nursing education to this day.

UC NURSING

In 2001, the college began offering international clinical opportunities to students to meet community health course requirements. The first destination was Honduras. The program has since expanded to Tanzania and Ecuador. Alumna Janet Johnson, who earned her bachelor's degree in nursing from the college in 1992, wanted to see more students have what she felt was a "life impacting" experience.

"Providing medical services in a Third World country, where even basic care can be lifesaving, is something all nurses should have the opportunity to experience," Johnson says. It's one of the main reasons she decided to establish a scholarship fund to assist with the College of Nursing's International Program.

While enrollments continued to increase, local health care facilities were still dealing with a nursing workforce shortage. The nursing vacancy rate at some facilities was above 20 percent. Yet again, this provided increased opportunity for students. Partnering with University of Cincinnati Medical Center, named University Hospital (UH) at the time, the college began offering a nursing co-op

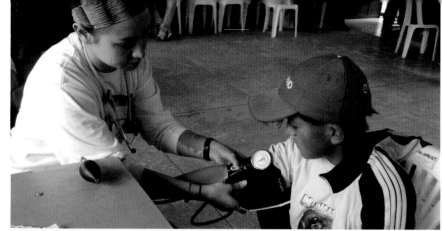

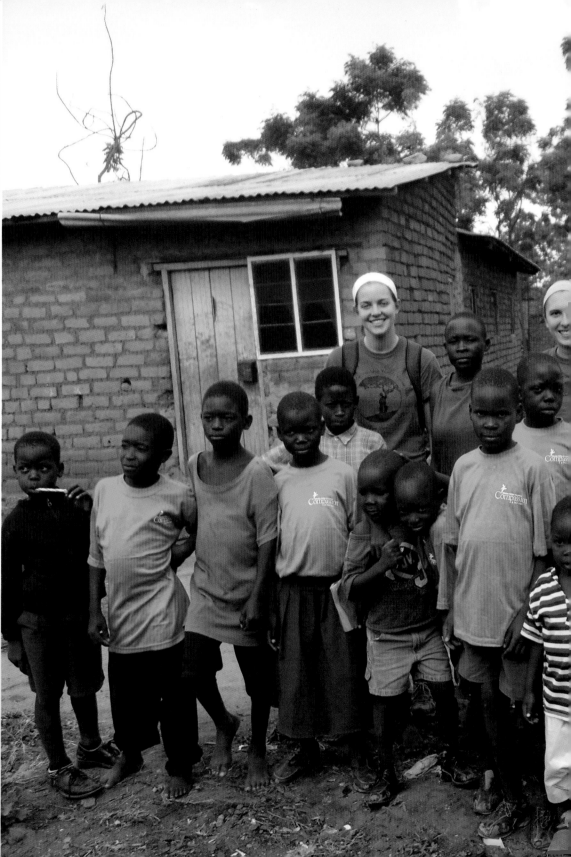

Top: Kelly Brown (BSN '12) takes a young boy's blood pressure.

Bottom: Quito, Ecuador; In 2008, nursing student Alex Freisthler (BSN '08) raised money for a year-long stay in Santa Lucia, Honduras, to practice nursing with Shoulder to Shoulder, a nonprofit health clinic. He was the clinic's first extended-stay nurse to come out of UC's College of Nursing. He was also the first long-term nurse with Shoulder to Shoulder. Shoulder to Shoulder was founded in 1996 by Jeff Heck, MD, a former professor at the UC College of Medicine who serves as the organization's executive director. The College of Nursing started collaborating with Shoulder to Shoulder in 2001.

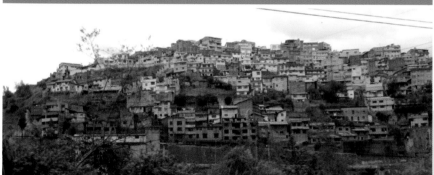

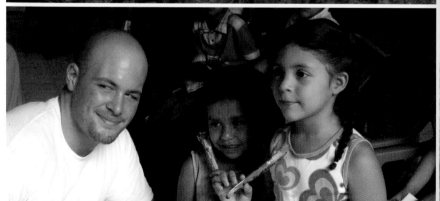

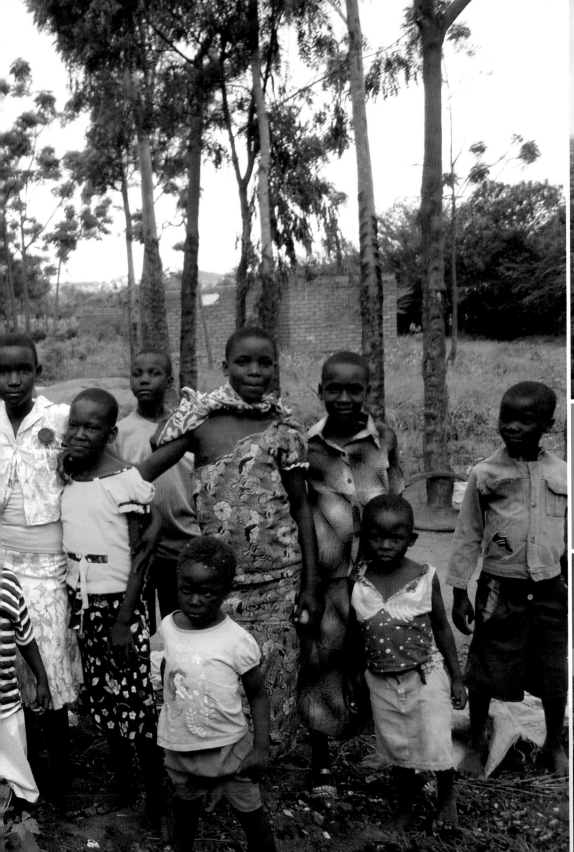

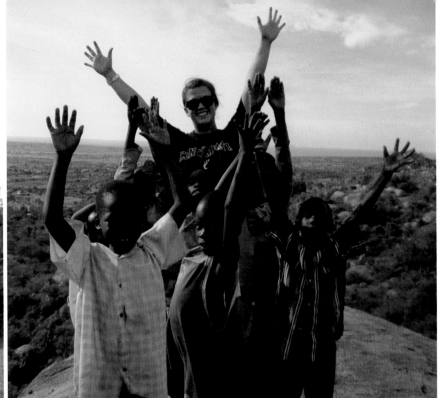

Top: Kelsey Dennis (BSN '12) poses with a group of children in Tanzania.
Middle: Mary Gsellman (BSN '12) and Kristen Henderson (BSN '12) take a group photo with local children in Tanzania.
Bottom: A delivery room in Tanzania.

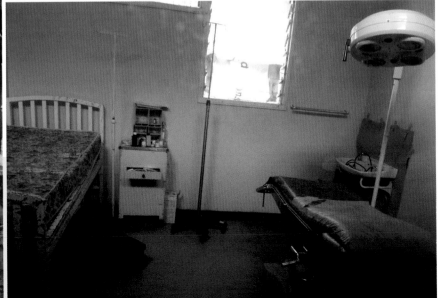

option to students. Karen Bankston, then vice president of operations at UH, and Carolyn Thomas, MSN, RN, then chief nursing officer at UH, partnered with the college to gain approval of the program by the State of Ohio Board of Nursing, as this was the first nursing co-op program offered in the state of Ohio. The co-op program had two goals:

- To provide additional opportunities for students to apply academic learning in a clinical setting, and
- To provide opportunity for potential recruitment of nursing students (to the organization).

The co-op program expanded to include other partner facilities, including Cincinnati Children's Hospital Medical Center. Students continue to have the opportunity to apply for this competitive program during their junior year of the BSN program.

WEDBUSH NURSING
Legacy Centre

In 2005, Jean Wedbush was visiting UC with her husband, Ed, a longtime member of UC's foundation board and College of Engineering alumnus. She decided to get some exercise by walking around the campus and stopped in the College of Nursing, where she met Lindell. That initial meeting led to a lasting friendship.

Wedbush, a nurse herself, became a significant supporter of the college. In 2007, the Wedbush Nursing Legacy Centre was opened as a result of

(Source for much of Chapter 12 material: Academic Health Center Public Relations and Communications.)

Jean and Ed's financial generosity. The Centre displays nursing uniforms, instruments and supplies from the past 125 years, allowing students to see the transformation of the nursing profession over the years.

In 2008, Wedbush received an honorary degree from the College of Nursing. She and her husband continue to be partners in the college's transformation and innovation initiatives.

2000-2009

2001 The college began offering international community health clinical opportunities to students. The first destination was Honduras.

2002 Students receive additional real world nursing experience at local hospitals. The college established the first Center for Aging with Dignity dedicated to promoting dignity, well-being and health for the aging and chronically ill.

2004 The first Center for the Scholarship of Teaching and Learning was established.

2005 The college offered its first distance learning programs. The Nurse Midwifery and Women's Health programs were offered completely online. The college's undergraduate program expanded as the first Clermont BSN cohort began studies at the Clermont Campus in Batavia, Ohio.

2007 The Wedbush Nursing Legacy Centre was established offering a space to showcase nursing history and memorabilia. This centre was generously made possible through a donation from Jean and Ed Wedbush.

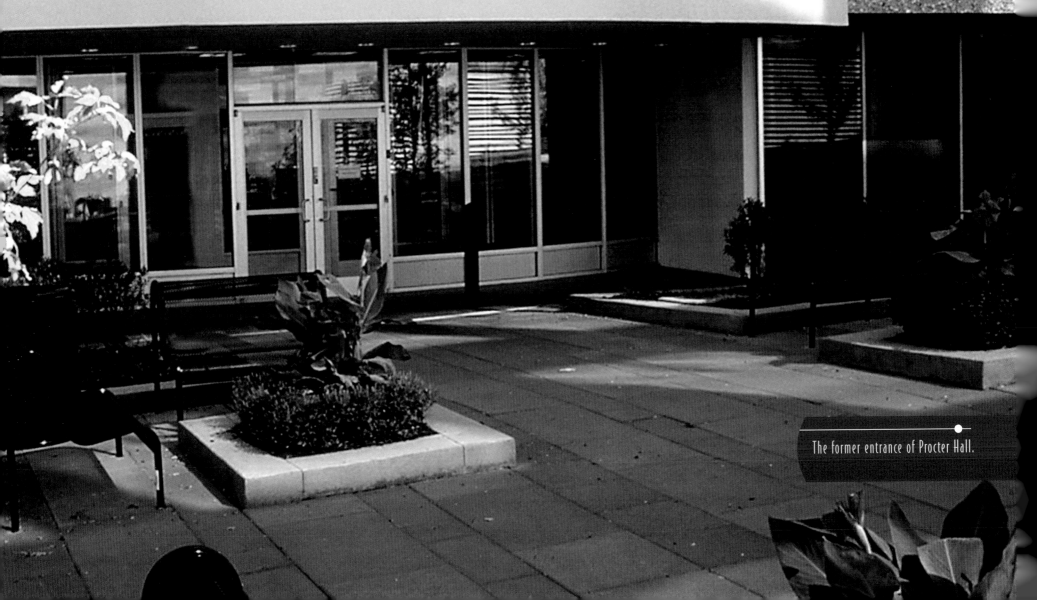

The former entrance of Procter Hall.

PAVING THE WAY TO THE FUTURE 2010–2014

Chapter Thirteen

Dean Andrea Lindell, PhD, RN, ANEF, announced her retirement from the college effective January 1, 2011, after 20 years in the position. Cheryl Hoying, PhD, RN, was named interim dean of the College of Nursing. Dr. Hoying had served as senior vice president of patient services at Cincinnati Children's Hospital Medical Center and, in 2007, was named associate dean of the College of Nursing. Starting in January 2011, she served as president of the American Organization of Nurse Executives.

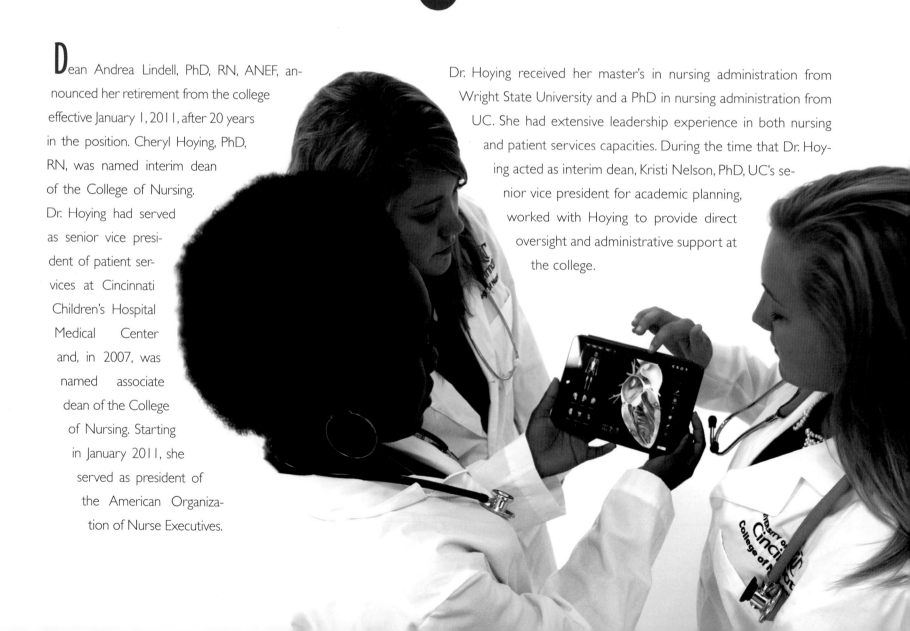

Dr. Hoying received her master's in nursing administration from Wright State University and a PhD in nursing administration from UC. She had extensive leadership experience in both nursing and patient services capacities. During the time that Dr. Hoying acted as interim dean, Kristi Nelson, PhD, UC's senior vice president for academic planning, worked with Hoying to provide direct oversight and administrative support at the college.

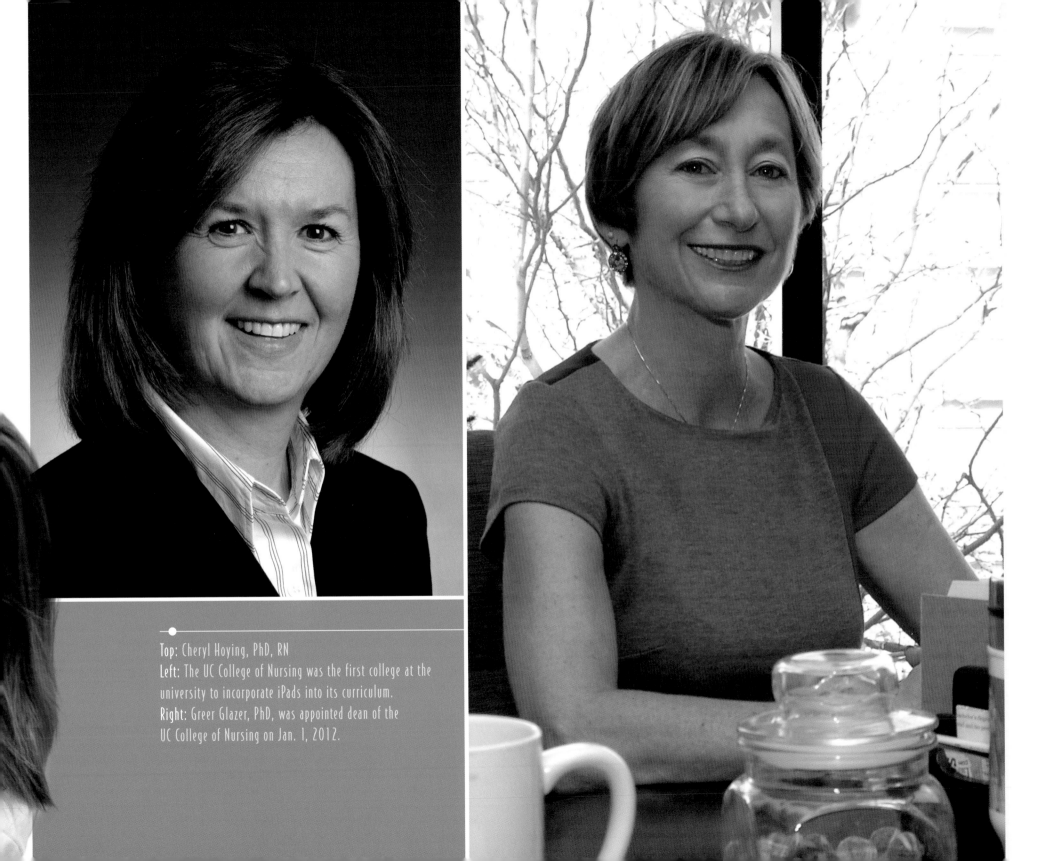

Top: Cheryl Hoying, PhD, RN
Left: The UC College of Nursing was the first college at the university to incorporate iPads into its curriculum.
Right: Greer Glazer, PhD, was appointed dean of the UC College of Nursing on Jan. 1, 2012.

Neville Pinto, PhD, dean of the UC Graduate School, chaired the search committee for the next nursing dean.

said Santa Ono, PhD, then senior vice president for academic affairs and provost. "I'm confident that Dr. Glazer's nursing, administrative

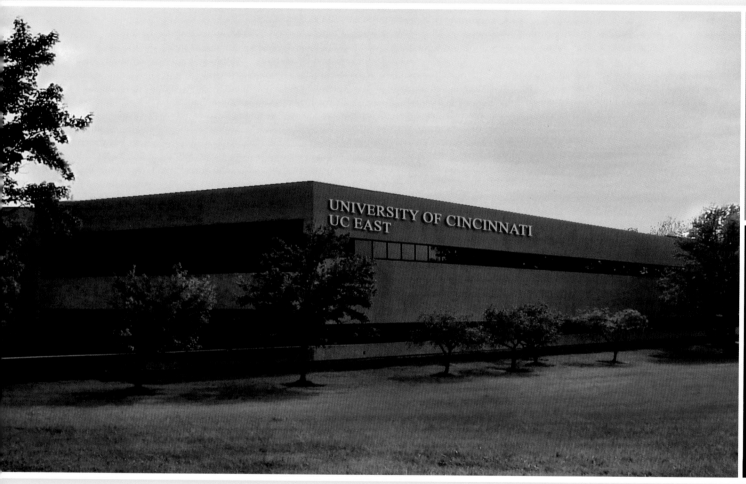

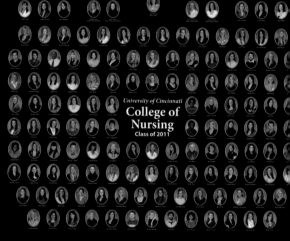

Left: The College of Nursing began offering the four-year bachelor of science in nursing program at UC East, a Clermont County expansion in the former Ford plant in Batavia Township.
Bottom: Class of 2011.
Right: Senior Associate Dean for Academic Affairs Suzanne Perraud, PhD

Greer Glazer, PhD, dean and professor of nursing at the University of Massachusetts Boston, College of Nursing and Health Sciences, was appointed dean of the College of Nursing, effective Jan. 1, 2012.

"The strength and rich history of UC's College of Nursing no doubt contributed to our ability to recruit someone of Dr. Glazer's caliber,"

and research expertise will be a great addition to the college and the university as a whole."

Glazer graduated *summa cum laude* with a bachelor's degree in nursing from the University of Michigan in 1976 and received her master's in nursing with a maternal/newborn focus from Case West-

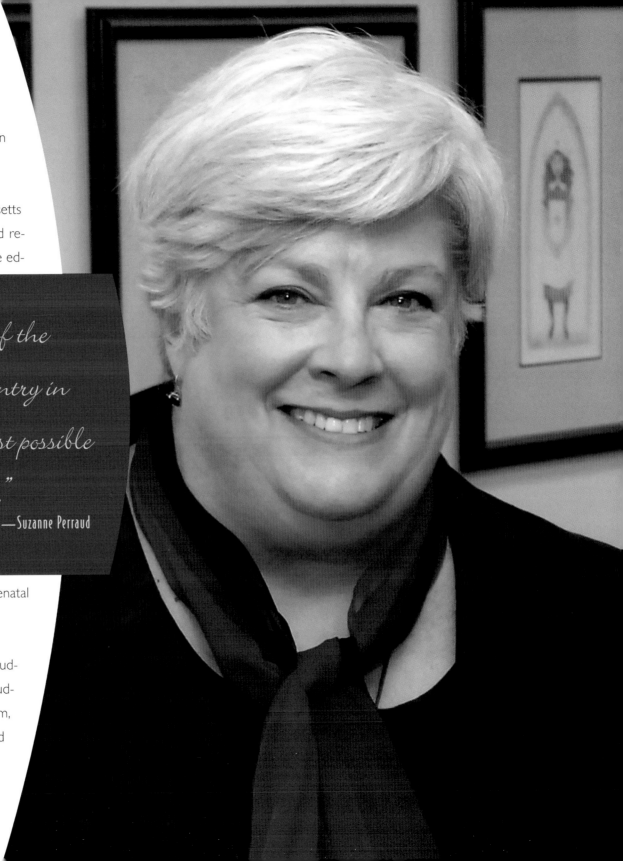

ern Reserve University in 1979. She received her PhD in nursing from Case Western in 1984. Glazer is also a Fulbright Scholar (in Israel '88) and a Robert Wood Johnson Executive Nurse Fellow 2001–04.

She held the dean's position at the University of Massachusetts from 2004 to 2011 and has extensive clinical, teaching and research experience, conducting studies on domestic violence ed-

"We are on our way to becoming one of the leading colleges of nursing in the country in leveraging technology to deliver the best possible classroom experience for our students."

—Suzanne Perraud

ucation, alcohol use during pregnancy and barriers to prenatal health care among African-American women.

Glazer's administrative responsibilities in Massachusetts included service or chairmanship on a number of committees, including the University Strategic Plan Implementation Design Team, the Chancellor's Strategic Planning Taskforce, Academic and Enrollment Planning Subcommittee and the Provost Search

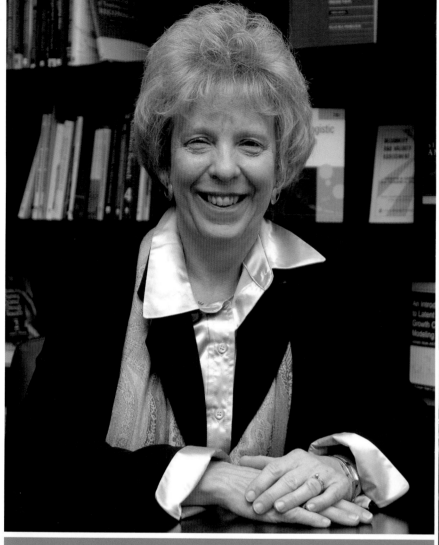

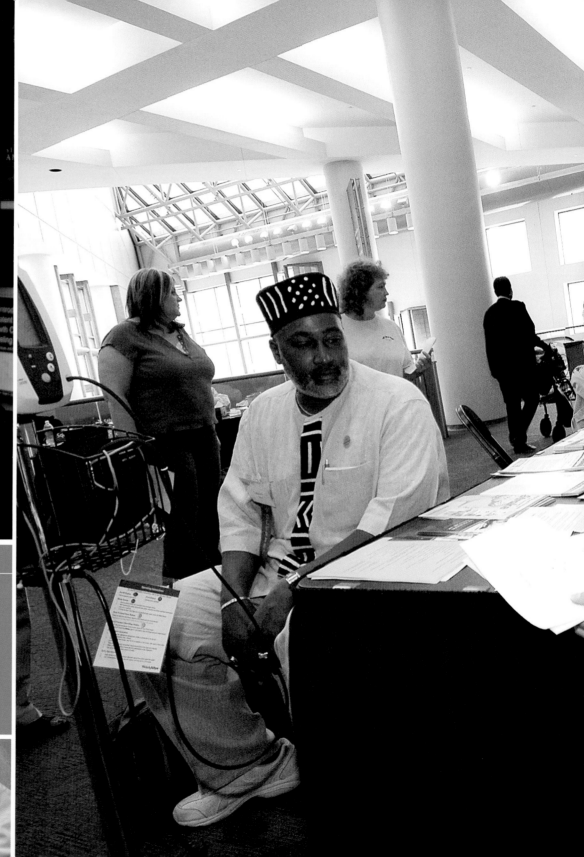

Top: Associate Dean of Research and Translation Donna Martsolf, PhD *(Dan Davenport)*

Bottom (left to right): A UCMC staff nurse assists a UC College of Nursing student; student simulation.

Right: UC College of Nursing student provides health screenings at a community event.

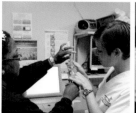

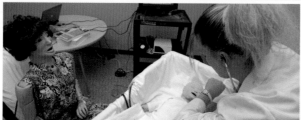

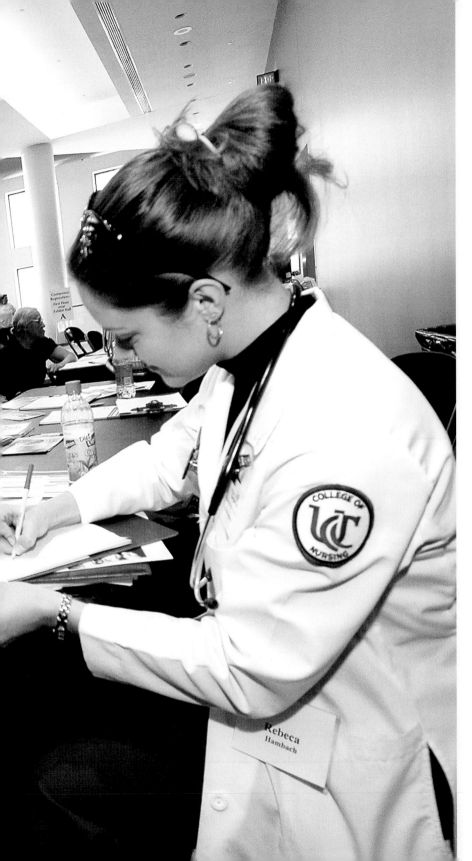

Committee, among many others. From 2007 to 2008 Glazer chaired the Urban Health and Public Policy Research Cluster Workgroup.

"I can't wait to join this vibrant community under the leadership of the visionary Provost and President," Glazer said, adding: "With the passage of the Affordable Health Care Act and the Institute of Medicine/Robert Wood Johnson Report on the Future of Nursing, I can't think of a better time to lead such an outstanding College of Nursing in curricular innovation, increased multidisciplinary and transdisciplinary research, community and global outreach, interprofessional education and academic service partnership."

> "I truly wanted to be a part of advancing the contribution of nursing in the improvement of health care in this region and beyond," says Martsolf.

Even before Dean Glazer got to Cincinnati, she started assembling her leadership team. Associate Dean for Research and Translation Donna Martsolf, PhD, came to the UC College of Nursing from Kent State University, where she served as a faculty member from 1993–2011. Dr. Glazer was also one of her colleagues at Kent State University in the 1990s.

"I caught Greer's vision for the college! We have very similar views on what the discipline of nursing is and how nurses can lead in health care. I also share her vision about the importance of leading in nursing education and in research. I truly wanted to be a part of advancing the contribution of nursing in the improvement of health care in this region and beyond," says Martsolf.

Dr. Martsolf adds, "I see us making great strides to advance the college strategic map. We truly are creatively leveraging technology to lead the transformation of health care in partnership, always informed by the people whom we serve. In the area of research we are recruiting and adding to our existing group of faculty members who conduct research in focused areas. Each year we add to the number of submitted and funded grants to advance our research endeavors. I am very pleased to be working with faculty, staff and students who are forming teams to conduct a variety of research projects that will improve the health and lives of the people we serve."

Senior Associate Dean for Academic Affairs Suzanne Perraud had also met Greer earlier.

"I was fortunate to have spent most of my career in a small but mighty college of nursing in Chicago at Rush University. I learned so much there and made many friends, one of whom introduced me to Dean Glazer," says Perraud, PMHCNS-BC, PhD. "The dean in turn seeded the idea of a move to Cincinnati. I was intrigued by the promise of what I could learn from applying the skills that I had developed in that small private school to a large and bustling college of nursing set in a public university. Aiding my decision was the fact that I had family in Cincinnati who warmly welcomed this Chicago transplant."

Dr. Perraud adds, "I see great things in the future for the College of Nursing at UC. We are on our way to becoming one of the leading colleges of nursing in the country in leveraging technology to deliver the best possible classroom experience for our students. The preparation of critical thinkers in nursing who can use data to solve problems and who understand the interprofessional nature of health care will set the stage for change in the workplace. And, I see the development of lasting partnerships with the rest of the Academic Health Center and with the world-class medical centers in our neighborhood, which will lead to the sharing of the best and brightest of our faculty and students to further lay the groundwork for the transformation of health care."

Dr. Karen Bankston, RN, AS, BSN, MSN, PhD, moved to Cincinnati many years ago. She was young, but not inexperienced. But when she got here, "I did a lot of growing up," she says. "Cincinnati is unbelievable. [It's] stuck in the past."

Bankston—the associate dean for Clinical Practice, Partnership and Community Engagement—has a long track record with health care in Cincinnati. She worked at (what was then called) The University Hospital and is the former CEO of Drake Center and the former Chief Nursing and Operations Officer at University of Cincinnati Medical Center. She received her PhD and was named CEO of the Drake Center within five days of each other: not a bad week. She was the first African American named as the CEO of a Cincinnati hospital—but there hasn't been one since.

Bankston is from Youngstown, a product of the public schools. She started school right after the Brown v. Board of Education decision.

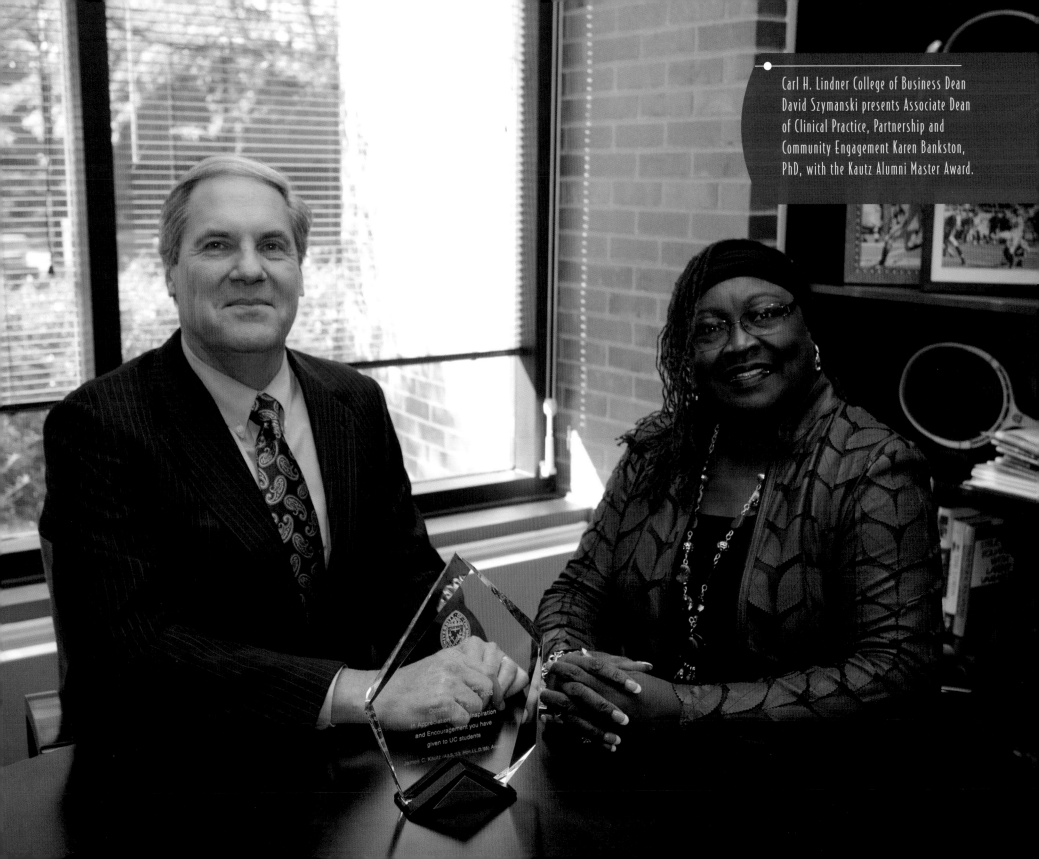

Carl H. Lindner College of Business Dean David Szymanski presents Associate Dean of Clinical Practice, Partnership and Community Engagement Karen Bankston, PhD, with the Kautz Alumni Master Award.

"Things have changed," she says. "I didn't know I was poor. My mom was a single mom. And I was embarrassed about that. Now when I hear kids say that they can't do it because they're poor, I'm [she shakes her head]…I don't know. There were other things going on back then that were harmful that left lifelong scars. Much of what's wrong now for kids is of their own doing."

"Now I have an opportunity to influence young minds while they're still fresh," Bankston says. "We are all a product of our experiences. [But] we have to learn to control our behaviors."

When Glazer first called Bankston to be part of a transformative team at the UC College of Nursing, Bankston's answer was immediate.

"I said, 'No.'" Bankston laughs at the memory. "I've known Greer for a long time—since the 80s and the Ohio Nursing Association and Public Policy Commission when Greer chaired it. She was just as much a firecracker back then as she is now in her old age!"

"That was 2011. Well, that same year I had just retired from being CEO of Drake Center to start my own consulting business, KDB & Associates. I focused on speaking to groups about change, process improvement, leadership development, inclusion and motivation. I gave a lot of speeches. I was also an adjunct in the College of Business teaching organizational leadership.

So there I was doing my thing, minding my own business. Greer comes to town and asks me to eat dinner with her."

"She says, 'I still want you.' I said, 'Tell me what you really need me to do.' She said she needed me to raise visibility in the health care arena, establish UC as a leader in the field, and partner with the appropriate players in the community."

"She invited me to meet the rest of the team. I came with some trepidation. I told them that as an alum—my PhD is from UC—I was disappointed. The state of health care is rapidly changing and I was disappointed that UC wasn't more visible in the dialogue. I said, 'Because I'm at the table and I don't see you guys there.' 'OK, we love you,' they said."

She is, so far, the only African American to graduate from the College of Nursing's PhD program. An African graduated, but no other African Americans.

"'Why have we graduated only one?' I ask," she says. "Others came through but didn't graduate." Right now, there's hope: there are African-American students in the pipeline.

Bankston is part of the team that applied for and received a grant from the Health Resources and Services Administration (HRSA—under the U.S. Department of Health and Human Services) "to expand the diversity at the college from historically marginalized populations for students who had potential but not the opportunity to go to college."

tion," she says. "The program calls for rigorous academic standards but also has a social component to it, too."

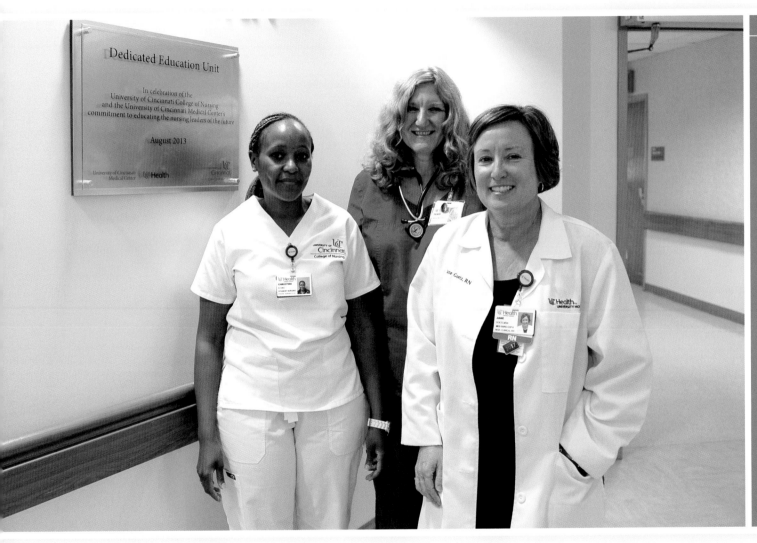

Left: In August 2013, the UC College of Nursing and University of Cincinnati Medical Center (UCMC) announced a partnership that established a Dedicated Education Unit (DEU) at UCMC. A DEU is a unique clinical teaching model and is an innovative way of providing clinical education to nursing students. Traditionally, nursing students go to a hospital as a group of approximately eight to 10 students with one faculty member. In the DEU model, a hospital unit hosts students from a single school of nursing, and staff nurses share in the clinical education of nursing students. Specifically, the DEU clinical education model is designed to give nursing students the best clinical experience available by pairing UCMC staff nurses one-on-one with individual junior UC nursing students through an entire term.
Middle: The DEU entrance at UCMC.

The college then works with students in 11th and 12th grade through sophomore year of college: "students who are on the bubble, who have the grades but not the ACT scores, maybe. The criteria include first gen, socioeconomic status, and being of a marginalized population.

"I have learned so much here. I believe I have brought much information and many skills to the college as well. I know this because I possessed a different skill set that was useful for transformation. I'm not an academician: I'm an operator," Bankston says. "It is God's plan that

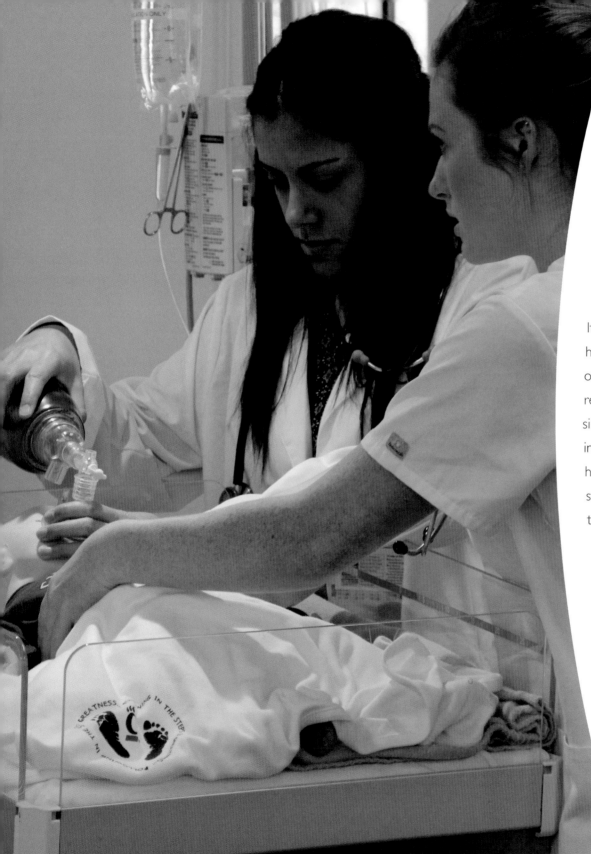

I'm here. Life is what you make it. God places you where he needs you to be when he needs you to be there."

The last recruit to join Dean Glazer's newly formed team was Chief Officer of Innovation and Entrepreneurship Debi Sampsel, DNP, MSN, BA, RN. Sampsel came to UC from the Nursing Institute of West Central Ohio, headquartered at Wright State University, where she was the executive director for seven years and later the commercialization manager.

It was in that capacity that Sampsel made a name for herself in the health care field as self-declared academic "techie" of sorts. Not only was she the principal investigator on the first faculty/student research study using a remote presence robot in a human patient simulation setting, but she also designed and implemented the Living Laboratory Smart Technology House: a high-tech, two-story house that models an intergenerational home environment, where students and health care professionals learn to care for patients in their own homes rather than in a hospital or nursing home setting.

"Greer's energy and passion for developing innovative, interprofessional active learning environments for students matched my expertise and desires for student-centric learning," says Sampsel. "I could tell she was a visionary leader who really understood how vital it was to embrace telehealth, human patient simulation and other technologies in order to prepare our students for the transformation of health care delivery."

Students practice simulated scenarios in the Innovation Collaboratory.

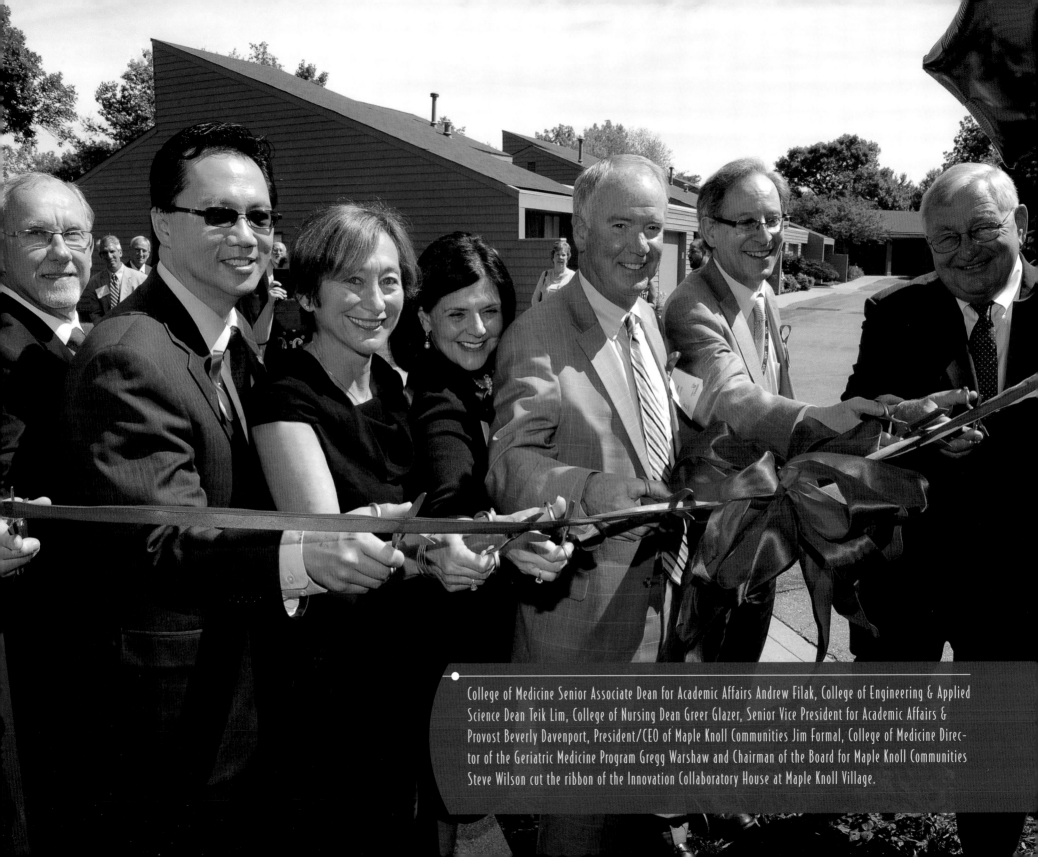

College of Medicine Senior Associate Dean for Academic Affairs Andrew Filak, College of Engineering & Applied Science Dean Teik Lim, College of Nursing Dean Greer Glazer, Senior Vice President for Academic Affairs & Provost Beverly Davenport, President/CEO of Maple Knoll Communities Jim Formal, College of Medicine Director of the Geriatric Medicine Program Gregg Warshaw and Chairman of the Board for Maple Knoll Communities Steve Wilson cut the ribbon of the Innovation Collaboratory House at Maple Knoll Village.

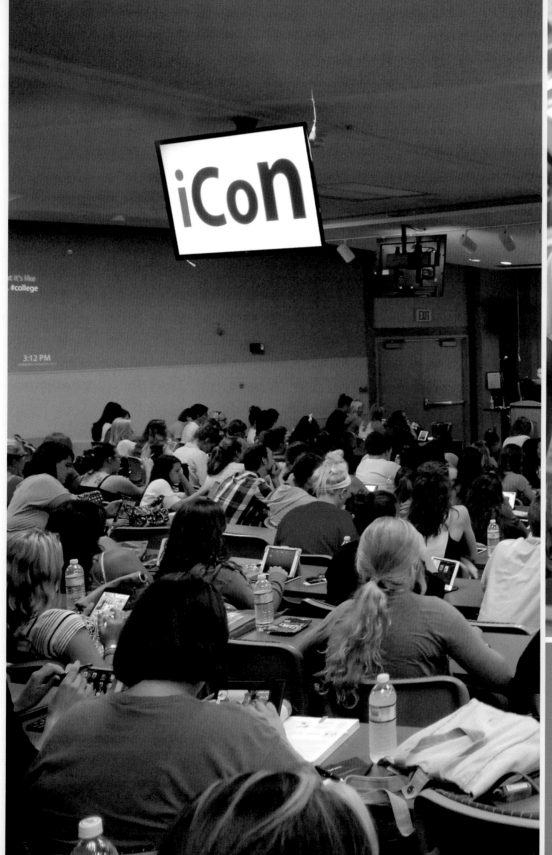

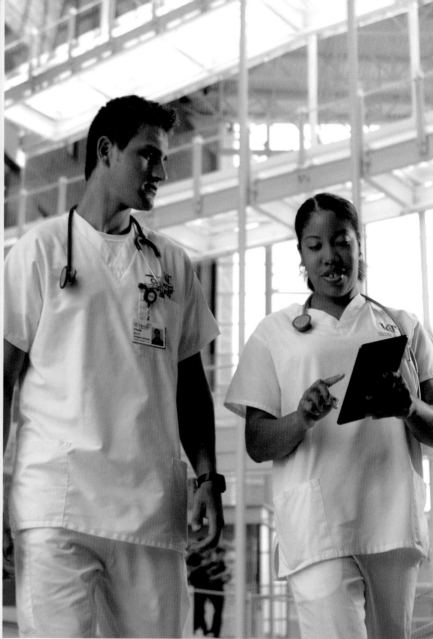

Top and left: In August 2013, the first class of sophomore nursing students went through an iPad orientation, called iCoN, to help them become acclimated to the college's new technology-based curriculum.

THE FUTURE OF NURSING IS

In a short amount of time, this extraordinary group of leaders propelled the college into several new developments and achievements.

"UC College of Nursing has been an important leader for the Coalition of Urban Serving Universities national effort to develop a health workforce that improves health and reduces health disparities in cities," said Jennifer Danek, MD, senior director of Urban Universities for HEALTH.

In October 2012, the University of Cincinnati was named one of five urban universities to participate in the Urban Universities for HEALTH learning collaborative, a national academic learning collaborative focused on investigating approaches to health care workforce development that lead to improved health outcomes and reduced disparities in local communities.

Urban Universities for HEALTH has awarded UC's Academic Health Center a four-year grant totaling more than $400,000 toward the research endeavor. The Academic Health Center comprises the colleges of Medicine, Nursing, Pharmacy and Allied Health Sciences and other programs and institutes on UC's medical campus.

"To be one of only five universities chosen is testament to where UC stands in academic excellence and dedication to best practices in health care," said Dean Greer Glazer, PhD, who co-wrote UC's grant proposal with Barbara Tobias, MD, Robert & Myfanwy Smith Endowed Professor, UC Department of Family and Community Medicine, and medical director of the Health Collaborative of Greater Cincinnati.

According to the Urban Universities for HEALTH, the collaborative is meant to engage top university and health professions leadership across disciplines in order to assess and improve institutional effectiveness, share information on what works and translate the knowledge into tools and resources for broader application.

One of the many ways that the College of Nursing is moving into the future is by putting technology into the hands of its students on a daily basis—literally. In 2013, starting with the sophomore class, course materials were delivered with an iPad for each student.

"Our integration of iPad represents a shift—a real opportunity to not just impact education, but to transform the way we learn, interact and collaborate," says Chris

Edwards, assistant vice president of e-learning, UCIT, and—at the time—assistant dean for information technology and communications and director of the Center for Academic Technology and Education Resources (CATER) at the College of Nursing. In 2013, Edwards was named an Apple Distinguished Educator by Apple.

Associate Professor Christine Colella, DNP, who was among the first faculty trained at the iPad Institute, is already using the audio feature of an application called Heart Murmur Pro to teach her Advanced Health Assessment and Differential Diagnosis classes. The application, she says, gives students the opportunity to hear over 23 different heartbeat sounds so they can discern which of the examples were indicative of an abnormal heart murmur.

"I think anything that engages the student makes for a better class," says Colella, who also uses Musculoskeletal Pro 3, which displays 10 layers of superficial and deep muscle with a 360-degree rotation of anatomic systems.

"The college will continue to develop unique transitional learning environments, similar to the Innovation Collaboratory Smart House, in order to mirror the evolving futuristic care delivery systems and to replicate 'real life experiences,'" says Debi Sampsel. "An intertwined technological and clinical pedagogy will produce highly masterful clinical and research oriented

nursing graduates who will be highly sought after by health care organizations across the country."

The students of today are looking forward to becoming nurses of the future, and that is what they are finding at the UC College of Nursing under Dean Glazer.

"The College of Nursing is committed to going wherever our students deserve to go!" says Assistant Dean of Student Affairs Krista Maddox, EdD. "Much freedom, responsibility and excitement comes with assuming a leading role in nursing education. Our students get to experience the benefits of cutting-edge curriculum and instruction that will make them sought-after practitioners."

An alum, former college administrator and now colleague in the Cincinnati health care community agrees.

"As a graduate of the University of Cincinnati College of Nursing, I saw first-hand the caliber of professionals who make the college thrive," says Cheryl Hoying, PhD, RN, NEA-BC, FACHE, FAAN, senior vice president, Patient Services at Cincinnati Children's Hospital Medical Center. "Today, in my role at Cincinnati Children's, I continually witness the results of the outstanding education the college provides nursing students. I am grateful that my association with the college continues—as former interim dean and currently as associate professor."

Chief Officer of Innovation and Entrepreneurship Debi Sampsel, DNP, MSN, BA, RN.

2010 ● The Doctor of Nursing Practice (DNP) program was approved by the Ohio Board of Regents in 2010, with admissions starting in fall 2010. The DNP curriculum is geared toward leadership, quality improvement, education and advanced practice.

2011 ● The college announced that it will offer all courses in the RN to BSN program online. The online RN to BSN program was developed to accommodate working adults who need to maintain their employment position while they are going to school.

2012 ● Online education and career information website SuperScholar.org named UC's College of Nursing as one of the Top 25 "Smart Choice" nursing schools for online nursing degrees.

The first eight students to graduate with a DNP from UC's College of Nursing were hooded June 9, 2012.

New Graduate Certificate in Nursing Education was offered for the first time.

2013 ● Dean Glazer was elected to the American Association of Colleges Nursing Board of Directors.

2014 ● College of Nursing began offering nurses a wider scope of advanced practice options to include two new postgraduate programs: a Psychiatric—Mental Health Nurse Practitioner (PMHNP) certificate and a Neonatal Nurse Practitioner (NNP).

The College of Nursing ranked No. 37 by *U.S. News & World Report* in its "2014 Best Online Programs" listing. The rankings—pulled from nearly 1,000 distance education programs surveyed—reflect scores from peer-to-peer evaluation, one-year retention rates, graduate rates and time required to graduate.

College held the "National Telehealth Conference: Transforming Health Care Delivery and Academic Curriculum." The objective of the National Telehealth Conference was to provide telehealth experiential learning for health care providers, administrators and faculty.

University of Cincinnati Innovation Collaboratory House opened on-site at Maple Knoll Village. This high-tech residence was developed—in partnership with Maple Knoll Village and UC's colleges of nursing, medicine and engineering and applied science—to determine whether technology can close the primary care gap for an aging population.

BIBLIOGRAPHY
Resources

Beckman, Wendy Hart. *Founders and Famous Families of Cincinnati.* Clerisy Press: 2014.

Cahall, Jean Brim, RN, BSN, MSN, PhD. *Pictorial History College of Nursing & Health 1889–1989 University of Cincinnati.* College of Nursing & Health Alumni Association, Cincinnati, Ohio: 1989.

Cangi, Ellen Corwin, PhD. "A New Profession for Women: The Art and Science of Nursing in Cincinnati, 1889–1940." *Queen City Heritage, The Journal of The Cincinnati Historical Society.* Volume 41, Winter 1983, Number 4, pp. 24–29.

Harlow, Alvin F. *The Serene Cincinnatians* (Society in America Series). New York: E. P. Dutton and Company, Inc., 1950.

Judd, Deborah M. "A New Century Brings Novel Ideas and Social Concerns." http://samples.jbpub.com/9780763759513/59513_chap5.pdf

Rosnagle, Laura, RN, and Mable I. Darrington, RN, "The Cincinnati University—A College of Nursing and Health." *Trained Nurse.* May 1950, pp. 217–247.

Venable, William Henry. *A Centennial History of Christ Church, Cincinnati: 1817–1917.* Stewart & Kidd Company, Cincinnati: 1918.

INDEX